Team-Based Care for Heart Failure

Editors

GREGG C. FONAROW
NANCY M. ALBERT

HEART FAILURE CLINICS

www.heartfailure.theclinics.com

Consulting Editors
MANDEEP R. MEHRA
JAVED BUTLER

Founding Editor
JAGAT NARULA

July 2015 • Volume 11 • Number 3

ELSEVIER

1600 John F. Kennedy Boulevard • Suite 1800 • Philadelphia, Pennsylvania, 19103-2899

http://www.theclinics.com

HEART FAILURE CLINICS Volume 11, Number 3
July 2015 ISSN 1551-7136, ISBN-13: 978-0-323-39100-9

Editor: Adrianne Brigido
Developmental Editor: Susan Showalter

Heart Failure Clinics (ISSN 1551-7136) is published quarterly by Elsevier Inc., 360 Park Avenue South, New York, NY 10010-1710. Months of publication are January, April, July, and October. Business and editorial offices: 1600 John F. Kennedy Boulevard, Suite 1800, Philadelphia, PA 19103-2899. Periodicals postage paid at New York, NY, and additional mailing offices. Subscription prices are USD 235.00 per year for US individuals, USD 382.00 per year for US institutions, USD 80.00 per year for US students and residents, USD 280.00 per year for Canadian individuals, USD 442.00 per year for Canadian institutions, USD 300.00 per year for international individuals, USD 442.00 per year for international institutions, and USD 100.00 per year for Canadian and foreign students/residents. To receive student and resident rate, orders must be accompanied by name of affiliated institution, date of term, and the *signature* of program/residency coordinator on institution letterhead. Orders will be billed at individual rate until proof of status is received. Foreign air speed delivery is included in all *Clinics* subscription prices. All prices are subject to change without notice. **POSTMASTER:** Send address changes to *Heart Failure Clinics*, Elsevier Health Sciences Division, Subscription Customer Service, 3251 Riverport Lane, Maryland Heights, MO 63043. **Customer Service: 1-800-654-2452 (US and Canada). From outside of the US and Canada, call 314-447-8871. Fax: 314-447-8029. For print support, E-mail: JournalsCustomerService-usa@elsevier.com. For online support, E-mail: JournalsOnlineSupport-usa@elsevier.com.**

Reprints. For copies of 100 or more of articles in this publication, please contact the Commercial Reprints Department, Elsevier Inc., 360 Park Avenue South, New York, NY 10010-1710. Tel.: 212-633-3874; Fax: 212-633-3820; E-mail: reprints@elsevier.com.

Heart Failure Clinics is covered in *MEDLINE/PubMed (Index Medicus).*

Contributors

CONSULTING EDITORS

MANDEEP R. MEHRA, MD, FACC, FACP, FRCP
Medical Director; Heart and Vascular Center and Executive Director, Center for Advanced Heart Disease; Brigham and Women's Hospital Professor of Medicine, Harvard Medical School, Boston, Massachusetts

JAVED BUTLER, MD, MPH
Professor of Medicine and Chief of Cardiology, Stony Brook University Heart Institute, Department of Internal Medicine, Stony Brook School of Medicine, Stony Brook University Medical Center, Stony Brook, New York

EDITORS

GREGG C. FONAROW, MD, FACC, FAHA
Professor of Medicine, Division of Cardiology, Department of Medicine; Director, Ahmanson-UCLA Cardiomyopathy Center, University of California, Los Angeles, California

NANCY M. ALBERT, PhD, CCNS, CHFN, CCRN, FAHA
Associate Chief Nursing Officer, Nursing Research and Innovation, Cleveland Clinic Health System and Clinical Nurse Specialist, Kaufman Center for Heart Failure, Cleveland Clinic Main Campus, Cleveland, Ohio

AUTHORS

LARRY A. ALLEN, MD, MHS
Division of Cardiology, Department of Medicine, University of Colorado School of Medicine, Aurora, Colorado

NAVEEN BELLAM, MD, MPH
Thomas Jefferson University, Philadelphia, Pennsylvania

TAMARA CHAKER, MSN
Division of Cardiology, Department of Medicine, Ahmanson-UCLA Cardiomyopathy Center, University of California, Los Angeles, California

LAUREN B. COOPER, MD
Fellow, Division of Cardiology, Department of Medicine, Duke Clinical Research Institute, Duke University School of Medicine, Durham, North Carolina

JULIE W. CREASER, MN
Division of Cardiology, Department of Medicine, Ahmanson-UCLA Cardiomyopathy

Center, University of California, Los Angeles, California

EUGENE C. DEPASQUALE, MD
Division of Cardiology, Department of Medicine, Ahmanson-UCLA Cardiomyopathy Center, University of California, Los Angeles, California

JOSIE DIMENGO, MSN, RN
Senior Liaison, Healthways, Inc, Employer Market, Franklin, Tennessee

MARY A. DOLANSKY, PhD, RN
Frances Payne Bolton School of Nursing, Case Western Reserve University, Cleveland, Ohio

STAVROS G. DRAKOS, MD, PhD
Department of Medicine, Division of Cardiology, University of Utah Health Sciences Center, Salt Lake City, Utah

JAMES C. FANG, MD
Division of Cardiology, University of Utah Health Sciences Center, Salt Lake City, Utah

TIMOTHY J. FENDLER, MD, MS
Division of Cardiovascular Outcomes Research, Saint Luke's Mid America Heart Institute, University of Missouri-Kansas City School of Medicine, Kansas City, Missouri

GREGG C. FONAROW, MD, FACC, FAHA
Professor of Medicine, Division of Cardiology, Department of Medicine; Director, Ahmanson-UCLA Cardiomyopathy Center, University of California, Los Angeles, California

PAUL HEIDENREICH, MD, MS
Professor and Vice-Chair, Department of Medicine, Stanford School of Medicine, Stanford, California; Cardiology, Palo Alto VA Medical Center, Palo Alto, California

ADRIAN F. HERNANDEZ, MD, MHS
Associate Professor of Medicine, Division of Cardiology, Department of Medicine, Duke Clinical Research Institute, Duke University School of Medicine, Durham, North Carolina

ANITA A. KELKAR, MD, MPH
Emory University School of Medicine, Atlanta, Georgia

PAUL M. LARSEN, MD
Resident Physician, Division of Internal Medicine, School of Medicine, University of California San Francisco, San Francisco, California

RITA McGUIRE, PhD, RN
Research Assistant Professor, University of Nebraska Medical Center, College of Nursing, Lincoln, Nebraska

JOSEPH NORMAN, PhD, PT
Professor, Division of Physical Therapy Education, University of Nebraska Medical Center, Omaha, Nebraska

BUNNY POZEHL, PhD, APRN-NP, FAHA, FAAN
Professor, University of Nebraska Medical Center, College of Nursing, Lincoln, Nebraska

MICHAEL W. RICH, MD
Professor, Division of Cardiology, Washington University School of Medicine, St Louis, Missouri

DARLENE ROURKE, MSN
Division of Cardiology, Department of Medicine, Ahmanson-UCLA Cardiomyopathy Center, University of California, Los Angeles, California

GERRYE STEGALL, MN, RN
Vice President, Healthways International, Franklin, Tennessee

KEITH M. SWETZ, MD, MA
Section of Palliative Medicine, Division of General Internal Medicine, Department of Medicine, Mayo Clinic, Rochester, Minnesota

JOHN R. TEERLINK, MD, FACC, FAHA, FESC, FRCP
Director, Heart Failure and Echocardiography, Section of Cardiology, San Francisco Veterans Affairs Medical Center; Professor of Medicine, School of Medicine, University of California San Francisco, San Francisco, California

JUDY TINGLEY, MPH, RN, AACC
Department of Surgery, Columbia University Medical Center, New York, New York

JUSTIN M. VADER, MD
Assistant Professor, Division of Cardiology, Washington University School of Medicine, St Louis, Missouri

ELIZABETH VANDENBOGAART, MSN
Division of Cardiology, Department of Medicine, Ahmanson-UCLA Cardiomyopathy Center, University of California, Los Angeles, California

MARY NORINE WALSH, MD, FACC
Department of Heart Failure and Cardiac Transplantation, St Vincent Heart Center of Indiana, Indianapolis, Indiana

OMAR WEVER-PINZON, MD
Department of Medicine, Division of Cardiology, New York-Presbyterian Hospital, Columbia University Medical Center, New York, New York

DAVID J. WHELLAN, MD, MHS
Professor of Medicine, Thomas Jefferson University, Philadelphia, Pennsylvania

Contents

There is substantial opportunity to reduce health care costs through prevention of heart failure. Team-based management of medical homes and large populations will be important for the success of any prevention interventions. Clinical trials of treatment are needed to show that heart failure is reduced by treatment. A team-based approach to treatment of asymptomatic left ventricular systolic dysfunction (LVSD) can work well with the availability of electronic medical records and a population approach to health. Attention should be given to optimizing risk factor reduction and preventive treatment with angiotensin-converting enzyme inhibitors/angiotensin receptor blockers and β-blockers if LVSD is present.

Hospitalizations for acute heart failure (HF) and subsequent readmissions have received increased attention because of the burden they place on patients, providers, and the health care system. These hospitalizations represent a significant portion of the total cost of HF care and health care in general. Although much of the care of the patient with HF occurs outside of the hospital, the genesis of the programs that attempt to limit repeat hospitalizations begin in the impatient setting. By using evidence-based guidelines, interdisciplinary teams, and comprehensive discharge planning, costly readmissions can be reduced and outcomes improved.

Transitions of care are a highly vulnerable period for patients living with heart failure. With the focus on increasing efficiencies and cost-effectiveness of the health care delivery system, clinicians are looking at models that have proved their effectiveness at improving the quality of care in this population. In this article, the changes in health care, frameworks for team-based approaches to care, and models of transitional care patient management that have been effective in other patient populations are examined.

Management of heart failure requires a multidisciplinary team-based approach that includes coordination of numerous team members to ensure guideline-directed optimization of medical therapy, frequent and regular assessment of volume status, frequent education, use of cardiac rehabilitation, continued assessment for the use of advanced therapies, and advance care planning. All of these are important aspects of the management of this complex condition.

Cardiovascular comorbidities have well-established relationships with morbidity and mortality indices in appropriately selected patients with heart failure. Caring for these conditions in current practice is no longer delivered by the sole general cardiologist, but rather by a network of health care providers. This article discusses the data supporting the management of cardiovascular comorbid conditions in heart failure, along with information highlighting the advantages of multidisciplinary care. Special attention is made regarding the role of affiliate providers and their impact in management of these conditions.

Heart failure (HF) treatment and prognosis are heavily influenced by the presence of noncardiac comorbid conditions. This article reviews the current evidence for the role of team-based care strategies to enhance care and improve outcomes in patients with HF with prevalent comorbidities. Few studies have evaluated the effects of team-based care on clinical and quality-of-life outcomes in patients with HF and specific comorbid conditions. Additional research is needed to clarify the impact and cost-effectiveness of team-based care for this population, particularly those patients with HF with multiple coexisting comorbid conditions.

Current guidelines of care recommend exercise in patients with stable chronic heart failure (HF); however, specifics of this exercise are not detailed. Cardiac rehabilitation for HF-reduced ejection fraction is now reimbursed by the Centers for Medicare and Medicaid, and many major insurance companies also reimburse cardiac rehabilitation irrespective of type or severity of HF. Although exercise-training guidelines and position statements are available for patients with HF, there has not been inclusion of HF disease management in core components or core competency statements for cardiac rehabilitation.

Telemonitoring for patients with heart failure has not become part of routine care; however it can have a place in multidisciplinary care planning, depending on the needs, goals and capabilities of patients and healthcare systems. Outcomes of clinical trials to date have been inconsistent in identifying the impact of telemonitoring on hospitalization and mortality. Studies incorporating self-care and behavior change theory with use of technology show promise. The abundance of new, portable technology that includes interactive features provides an opportunity to study device effectiveness in promoting and monitoring heart failure self-care and develop best-practice strategies. This article will address the findings of previous studies and provide recommendations for future consideration.

Advanced heart failure (AHF) is the end stage of the heart failure syndrome that is associated with significant morbidity, high mortality, and rising costs that pose a significant burden for the different health care systems in the United States and worldwide. Despite advances in pharmacologic and device therapy, patients with AHF frequently require complex therapies, such as continuous infusion of inotropic agents, mechanical circulatory support, and heart transplant. This article summarizes the team-based approach to care of patients with AHF and those supported by left ventricular assist devices.

Clinical practice guidelines endorse the use of palliative care in patients with symptomatic heart failure. Palliative care is conceptualized as supportive care afforded to most patients with chronic, life-limiting illness. However, the optimal content and delivery of palliative care interventions remains unknown and its integration into existing heart failure disease management continues to be a challenge. Therefore, this article comments on the current state of multidisciplinary care for such patients, explores evidence supporting a team-based approach to palliative and end-of-life care for patients with heart failure, and identifies high-priority areas for research.

Team-based or multidisciplinary care may be a potential way to positively impact outcomes for heart failure (HF) patients by improving clinical outcomes, managing patient symptoms, and reducing costs. The multidisciplinary team includes the HF cardiologist, HF nurses, clinical pharmacists, dieticians, exercise specialists, mental health providers, social workers, primary care providers, and additional subspecialty providers. The timing and setting of multidisciplinary care depends on the needs of the patient and the resources available. Multidisciplinary HF teams should be evaluated based on their ability to achieve goals, as well as their potential for sustainability over time.

Foreword

The Winning Team in Heart Failure: Dimensionality of Care Redesign

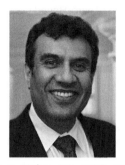
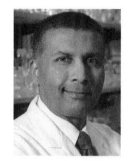

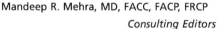

Mandeep R. Mehra, MD, FACC, FACP, FRCP   Javed Butler, MD, MPH

Consulting Editors

> *There is no 'i' in team but there is in win*
> —*Michael Jordan*

The editors of this issue of *Heart Failure Clinics*, the dream team of Drs Gregg Fonarow and Nancy Albert, exemplify the need for developing winning partnerships in redesigning heart failure care across the spectrum of disease severity and comorbidity. Chronic heart failure care necessitates development of care paradigms that must take a holistic view of the patient's disease well beyond the frequent episodes of care. We believe that a well-refined approach to care must take three dimensions into account as care plans are developed, including (1) the patient's disease status and control of its elements; (2) care of modifiable and nonmodifiable comorbidities; and (3) psychosocial and biobehavioral barriers to care. Unless these multiple dimensions are accounted for, care plans to address the natural history of the disease trajectory will likely fall short.

To drive home this point, we must remember that the typical heart failure patient is now elderly and frail, suffers from cognitive difficulties and surrounding comorbidities, and consumes a panoply of medications. Reciprocal associations between heart failure and comorbidities exist for practically all body organ systems, including chronic obstructive lung disease, liver disease, chronic kidney disease, skeletal myopathy, anemia, multiple endocrine disorders, including, particularly, diabetes mellitus and thyroid disorders, as well as psychological disorders, including depression and anxiety. Each of these facets is particularly prevalent and similarly difficult to manage in the archetypical elderly heart failure patient.

Thus, it really does take a village to take care of these patients in the best possible way. In this respect, the collaborative team-based approach of general medical and nursing practitioners with specialists of various backgrounds is obvious. However, what needs to be emphasized is that systems of care are needed to optimize patient outcomes that go beyond the doctor–nurse teams. Physical therapists, pharmacists, social workers, and other medical and paramedical personnel need to understand the special needs of this demanding patient population. Increasingly, palliative care interventions are important to address early in the course of disease in this syndrome.

Besides generic heart failure management, there are specific scenarios that necessitate strong consideration for team-based management. Starting at one end of the spectrum is prevention of heart failure that requires identification

Heart Failure Clin 11 (2015) ix–x
http://dx.doi.org/10.1016/j.hfc.2015.05.002
1551-7136/15/$ – see front matter © 2015 Published by Elsevier Inc.

and surveillance of high-risk patients and optimal risk-factor management. At the other end of the spectrum are patients with advanced heart failure, patients who require consideration for either advanced therapies like mechanical circulatory support or cardiac transplantation. These aspects of advanced heart failure require a unique form of advanced teams with "super specialization" in technology- and immunology-based approaches.

As technology advances, the importance of team-based management amplifies. There continue to be important advances in temporary and permanent mechanical circulatory support. Nonsurgical management of coronary and valvular heart diseases continues to evolve. All of these require collaboration between not only medical personnel but also biomedical engineers. Arguably, the most robust example of technological evolution is the growing field of telemonitoring that now allows the possibility of continuous 24-hour data on cardiac hemodynamics and rhythm that has necessitated the need for a collaborative management paradigm.

Perhaps no other part in the journey of patients with chronic heart failure exemplifies the importance of team-based care more than episodes of heart failure–related hospitalization. These patients are at an extraordinarily high risk of adverse outcomes. Importantly, they are cared for by a variety of cardiovascular and noncardiovascular medical specialists from emergency room presentation to discharge. Chronic medication and dietary patterns are altered. In an increasing number of cases in the modern health care delivery paradigm, the outpatient physicians are not involved in the management of these hospital episodes, despite the related elevated risk for short-term readmission and hospitalization. Transitions of care from inpatients to outpatients and the subsequent few months represent a particularly vulnerable phase. The Medicare readmission penalties for heart failure readmissions have further highlighted the importance of the team-based approach to optimize transitions of care to reduce the risk of readmissions.

These dynamics amply underscore the importance of this issue of *Heart Failure Clinics*, titled simply and precisely, "Team-Based Care for Heart Failure." Guest editors Drs Fonarow and Albert have assimilated an extraordinary group of experienced thought-leaders to give their perspectives on team-based management of heart failure across the spectrum of disease manifestation and care options. This issue is critical for optimal management of this complex group of patients, for medical professionals as well as for nonmedical professionals and administrators involved in heart failure care.

Mandeep R. Mehra, MD, FACC, FACP, FRCP
Heart and Vascular Center
Center for Advanced Heart Disease
Brigham and Women's Hospital
Harvard Medical School
75 Francis Street, A Building
3rd Floor, Room AB324
Boston, MA 02115, USA

Javed Butler, MD, MPH
Stony Brook University Heart Institute
Department of Internal Medicine
Stony Brook School of Medicine
Stony Brook University Medical Center
101 Nicolls Rd, Stony Brook, NY 11794, USA

E-mail addresses:
MMEHRA@partners.org (M.R. Mehra)
Javed.Butler@stonybrookmedicine.edu (J. Butler)

Preface

Team-based Care for Heart Failure

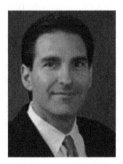 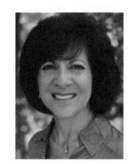

Gregg C. Fonarow, MD, FACC, FAHA   Nancy M. Albert, PhD, CCNS, CHFN, CCRN, FAHA

Editors

Heart failure remains a major public health problem, affecting over 5 million patients in the United States and over 23 million patients worldwide. Heart failure results in unacceptably high morbidity, mortality, and health care expenditures. The lifetime risk of developing heart failure is 1 in 5 for both men and women at the age of 40, and the incidence is nearly 10 per 1000 for men and women over the age of 65. Heart failure is the leading cause of hospitalization for persons 65 years of age, and rates of hospital readmission within 30 days are 20% to 25%. Heart failure also poses a substantial economic burden with annual direct costs for care of heart failure in the United States estimated to be between $31 and $60 billion. The personal burden of heart failure includes debilitating symptoms, functional limitations, frequent hospitalizations, and high rates of mortality. Optimal use of guideline-directed therapies, education, support, and involvement of patients with heart failure and their families is critical and often complex. Many overburdened clinicians have not fully integrated the evidence-based treatments recommended in heart failure guidelines into routine clinical practice. Failure of patients to understand and follow a detailed and often nuanced plan of care also contributes to the high rates of hospitalization, rehospitalization, and mortality seen with heart failure.

Care for patients with heart failure ideally integrates inpatient and outpatient health care delivery with goals of reducing symptoms, improving health status, increasing functional capacity, decreasing the need for hospitalization, and prolonging life. There has been tremendous interest regarding team-based care for heart failure in achieving these goals. Team-based care for prevention and treatment of heart failure may be organized in a variety of ways. Teams may consist of heart failure cardiologists, primary care physicians, advance practice nurses, home care nurses, cardiac rehabilitation clinicians, pharmacists, dieticians, medical social workers, care coordinators, health educators, and palliative care specialists. It is guideline-recommended that effective systems of care coordination be deployed for every patient with heart failure that facilitate and ensure effective care that is designed to achieve guideline-directed therapies and prevent hospitalization. Team-based care for heart failure can help facilitate a clear, detailed, and evidence-based plan of care that ensures the achievement of guideline-directed medical therapy goals, effective management of comorbid conditions, timely follow-up with the health care team, appropriate dietary and physical activities, and compliance with secondary prevention guidelines for cardiovascular disease. Team-based care can also help to ensure the heart failure plan of care is

Heart Failure Clin 11 (2015) xi–xii
http://dx.doi.org/10.1016/j.hfc.2015.05.001
1551-7136/15/$ – see front matter © 2015 Published by Elsevier Inc.

heartfailure.theclinics.com

updated regularly and available to all members of each patient's health care team. Multidisciplinary team-based heart failure disease-management programs are class I recommended for patients at high risk for hospital readmission, to facilitate the implementation of guideline-directed therapy, to address different barriers to behavioral change, and to reduce the risk of subsequent rehospitalization for heart failure.

This issue of *Heart Failure Clinics* is focused on the role of team-based care for heart failure. Prevention of heart failure (and preventing progression of heart failure) requires maintenance of multiple factors, from nutrition, weight, smoking, and other modifiable habits to treatment of cardiac and noncardiac diseases and control of dysrhythmias. Since preventive factors may be diverse, a healthy lifestyle, personal responsibility, and a team-based approach are essential to success. During hospitalization for acute decompensated heart failure and the transition period from hospital to home, patients are vulnerable to rehospitalization due to pathophysiologic, medical-management, sociocultural, psychological, and other factors. A team-based approach that includes assessment and outpatient management of the complexities of heart failure, cardiac and noncardiac conditions, aging, deconditioning, and other factors provides the best chance of delivery of and adherence to guideline-directed medical therapies. In this issue, team-based care is discussed in relation to prevention, hospitalization, transitions of care, outpatient management, and managing cardiac and noncardiac conditions.

Despite the effectiveness of self-care management behaviors on clinical outcomes, availability and reimbursement of cardiac rehabilitation to increase self-efficacy for activity and exercise, and external telemonitoring to increase awareness of new or worsening signs and symptoms of worsening condition, patient adherence to self-care may be inconsistent and nonoptimal. Articles on cardiac rehabilitation/exercise training and external telemonitoring outline barriers to use of available resources that limit benefits.

The diagnosis of advanced heart failure, and continued symptoms despite optimization of guideline-directed medical therapies, places a burden of caring on patients, families, and health care providers. In addition, frailty, depression, and cognitive dysfunction may be unrecognized and affect decision-making and self-care management. Patient-centered, multiprofessional care may enable communication on prognosis and goal adjustment that includes ventricular-assist device placement and management, discussions of advance directives, and palliative and end-of-life care. Interventions that support caregivers are needed, and more research is needed to determine the optimal time to start palliative interventions. Articles on team-based management of advanced heart failure and palliative and end-of-life care reinforce the need for coordinated care.

Finally, gaps and disparities in hospital and ambulatory heart failure access and care are well documented. Quality heart failure care cannot be presumed; rather, ongoing monitoring is needed to assure patients receive value-based care. Two articles in this issue discuss equitable heart failure care and assess the quality of comparative effectiveness of team-based care. It is our hope that this information proves useful in advancing the prevention and treatment of heart failure and helps guide future research into team-based care.

Gregg C. Fonarow, MD, FACC, FAHA
Division of Cardiology
Department of Medicine
Ahmanson-UCLA Cardiomyopathy Center
University of California
10833 LeConte Avenue
Room A2-237 CHS
Los Angeles, CA 90095, USA

Nancy M. Albert, PhD, CCNS, CHFN, CCRN, FAHA
Cleveland Clinic Health System
Mail Code J3-4
9500 Euclid Avenue
Cleveland, OH 44195, USA

E-mail addresses:
gfonarow@mednet.ucla.edu (G.C. Fonarow)
ALBERTN@ccf.org (N.M. Albert)

Heart Failure Prevention and Team-based Interventions

Paul Heidenreich, MD, MS[a,b]

KEYWORDS

- Heart failure • Intervention • Prevention • Cardiac

KEY POINTS

- There is substantial opportunity to reduce health care costs through prevention of heart failure.
- Team-based management of medical homes and large populations will be important for the success of any prevention interventions.
- Clinical trials of treatment are needed to show that heart failure is reduced by treatment.
- A team-based approach to treatment of asymptomatic left ventricular systolic dysfunction (LVSD) can work well with the availability of electronic medical records and a population approach to health.
- Attention should be given to optimizing risk factor reduction and preventive treatment with angiotensin-converting enzyme inhibitors/angiotensin receptor blockers and β-blockers if LSVD is present.

The prevalence of heart failure is expected to increase markedly during the next 20 years with the aging of the population of many Western countries. By 2030 it is expected that more than 8 million people in the United States will have heart failure (**Fig. 1**) unless the health care system can identify and implement effective preventive strategies.[1] The cost of caring for the growing number of patients with heart failure is expected to reach $160 billion per year (in today's dollars) by 2030 (**Fig. 2**). The potential cost savings are better reflected by the incremental costs caused by heart failure because patients will continue to be treated for other conditions if heart failure can be prevented. The cost analysis by the American Heart Association suggests that the incremental cost caused by heart failure will still be $58 billion by 2030.[1] Thus, there is substantial opportunity to reduce health care costs through prevention of heart failure. Team-based management of medical homes and larger populations will be important for the success of any prevention interventions.

STAGES OF HEART FAILURE

The American College of Cardiology (ACC) and American Heart Association (AHA) have described 4 stages of heart failure (A–D).[2] Stage A includes patients with only risk factors for heart failure. Stage B patients have structural heart changes but no symptoms. Typically these are defined as asymptomatic systolic dysfunction, diastolic dysfunction, left ventricular hypertrophy, and valve disease. Patients with heart failure symptoms are placed in stage C and those with end-stage disease are in stage D. To prevent heart failure (stages C and D), then patients must be targeted at either stage A or B. Depending on the risk factor, the time to develop heart failure has varied from 3 to 16 years (**Fig. 3**).[3] Given the several-year period

[a] Department of Medicine, Stanford School of Medicine, Stanford, CA 94305, USA; [b] Cardiology, Palo Alto VA Medical Center, 111C, 3801 Miranda Avenue, Palo Alto, CA 94304, USA
E-mail address: heiden@stanford.edu

Heart Failure Clin 11 (2015) 349–358
http://dx.doi.org/10.1016/j.hfc.2015.03.001
1551-7136/15/$ – see front matter Published by Elsevier Inc.

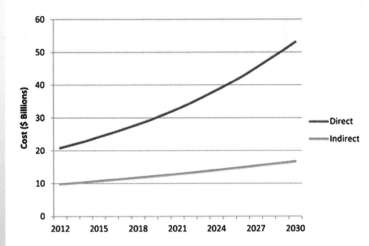

Fig. 1. The American Heart Association projected increase in US prevalence of heart failure to 2030. (*From* Heidenreich PA, Albert NM, Allen LA, et al, American Heart Association Advocacy Coordinating Committee, Council on Arteriosclerosis, Thrombosis and Vascular Biology, Council on Cardiovascular Radiology and Intervention, Council on Clinical Cardiology, Council on Epidemiology and Prevention, Stroke Council. Forecasting the impact of heart failure in the United States: a policy statement from the American Heart Association. Circ Heart Fail 2013;6:609; with permission.)

that usually occurs between heart failure stages it is possible that screening for modifiable characteristics will be helpful.

MODIFIABLE RISK FACTORS FOR HEART FAILURE (STAGE A)

Several modifiable risk factors for heart failure have been identified, including physical inactivity, cigarette smoking, obesity, diabetes, and hypertension.[4] These direct risk factors, along with hyperlipidemia, also contribute to coronary heart disease, which is itself a risk factor and may contribute to 60% of heart failure in the United States.[4] A more recent analysis attributed 53% of heart failure to these risk factors, with 20% caused by coronary disease; 20% to hypertension; and 13% split among smoking, obesity, and diabetes.[3] The mean number of risk factors per person was 1.9 ± 1.1 (out of 5).[3] Other risk factors are difficult (limited education) or impossible to modify (male sex).[4]

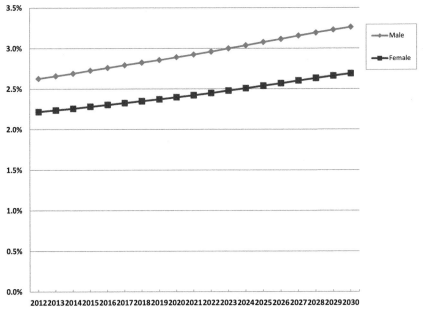

Fig. 2. The expected increase in cost of heart failure care to 2030 per the American Heart Association. This analysis avoids double counting of costs and is limited to the incremental costs caused by heart failure. (*From* Heidenreich PA, Albert NM, Allen LA, et al, American Heart Association Advocacy Coordinating Committee, Council on Arteriosclerosis, Thrombosis and Vascular Biology, Council on Cardiovascular Radiology and Intervention, Council on Clinical Cardiology, Council on Epidemiology and Prevention, Stroke Council. Forecasting the impact of heart failure in the United States: a policy statement from the American Heart Association. Circ Heart Fail 2013;6:606–19; with permission.)

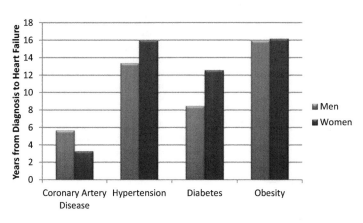

Fig. 3. The time delay between diagnosis of risk factor and onset of heart failure for the most common factors. (*Data from* Dunlay SM, Weston SA, Jacobsen SJ, et al. Risk factors for heart failure: a population-based case-control study. Am J Med 2009;122:1023–8.)

Hypertension

Hypertension is the most common risk factor and has been increasing over time among patients with heart failure.[3] It was present in 66% of patients during 1985 to 1990 and 74% from 1997 to 2002.[3] The effect of hypertension treatment on the development of heart failure has been evaluated in several clinical trials. A network meta-analysis[5] showed that diuretics (odds ratio [OR], 0.59 for development of heart failure), angiotensin-converting enzyme (ACE) inhibitors (OR, 0.70), and angiotensin II receptor blockers (OR, 0.76) were the most effective drugs in reducing the incidence of heart failure compared with placebo (**Fig. 4**). These drugs were more effective than calcium antagonists, β-blockers, and α-blockers (see **Fig. 4**). A separate meta-analysis evaluating the effect of β-blockers found that the degree of blood pressure reduction was the main determinant of success in reducing subsequent heart failure.[6] β-Blockers did not have a significant effect at reducing heart failure beyond blood pressure reduction.

Diabetes

Diabetes has been increasing among patients diagnosed with heart failure. In a population study from Rochester, Minnesota, diabetes was present in 13% of newly diagnosed patients with heart failure during 1985 to 1990 which increased to 21% from 1997 to 2002 (*P* = .003 for trend).[3] The time from onset of diabetes to the development of heart failure ranged from 8.5 years for men to 12.6 years for women.[3] In this study from Rochester, Minnesota, the population attributable risk of diabetes for incident heart failure was 12% (**Fig. 5**).

Smoking

Current or past smoking among patients with incident heart failure has increased slightly from 52% of newly diagnosed patients with heart failure during 1985 to 1990 to 58% during 1997 to 2002 (*P* = .001 for trend).[3] In the Women's Health Initiative the incidence of heart failure increased from 1.75 per 1000 person-years for never smokers to 2.01 for past smokers and to 3.33

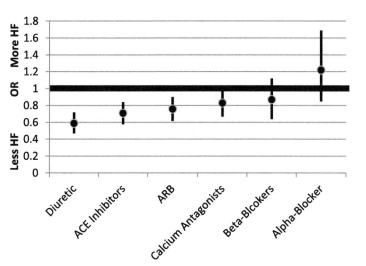

Fig. 4. The population attributable risk is shown for the different risk factors. For men, the most important risk factor is coronary artery disease, whereas for women it is hypertension. HF, heart failure. (*Data from* Dunlay SM, Weston SA, Jacobsen SJ, et al. Risk factors for heart failure: a population-based case-control study. Am J Med 2009;122:1023–8.)

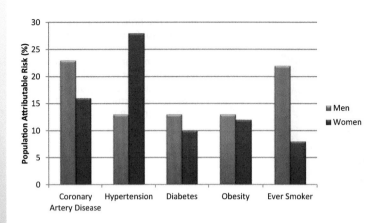

Fig. 5. Change in prevalence of risk factors over time. (*Data from* Huffman MD, Capewell S, Ning H, et al. Cardiovascular health behavior and health factor changes (1988–2008) and projections to 2020: results from the National Health and Nutrition Examination Surveys. Circulation 2012;125:2595–602; and *Courtesy of* NHANES (National Health and Nutrition Examination Survey).)

for current smokers.[7] After adjustment for other risk factors, the risk of incident heart failure for never smokers was 0.42 (95% confidence interval [CI], 0.35–0.49) and 0.52 (95% CI, 0.44–0.62) for past smokers compared with current smokers.[7] The average population attributable risk for ever smoking was 14%, ranging from 8% for women to 22% for men.[3]

Obesity

Obesity has been increasing among patients diagnosed with heart failure. In a population study from Rochester, Minnesota, obesity was present in 20.5% of newly diagnosed patients with heart failure during 1985 to 1990 compared with 29.5% from 1997 to 2002 (P = .003 for trend).[3] The average time from onset of obesity to the development of heart failure was 16 years.[3] The population attributable risk of obesity for incident heart failure was 12%. In a study from the Women's Health Initiative, the incidence of heart failure increased from 1.32 per 1000 person-years for patients with a body mass index (BMI) between 18.5 and 25 kg/m^2, to 1.72 per 1000 person-years for those with a BMI between 25 and 30 kg/m^2, and 3.37 per 1000 person-years for those with a BMI greater than 30 kg/m^2.[7] After adjustment for other risk factors, the risk developing heart failure for patients with a BMI between 18.5 and 25 kg/m^2 was 0.43 (95% CI, 0.38–0.48), and 0.50 (95% CI, 0.45–0.56) for those with a BMI between 25 and 30 kg/m^2 compared with those with a BMI greater than 30 kg/m^2.[7]

Physical Activity

In the Women's Health Initiative the incidence of heart failure ranged from 1.55 per 1000 person-years for physically active individuals (defined as ≥150 min/wk of moderate physical activity, or ≥75 min/wk of vigorous physical activity) to 2.15

for those who were somewhat active (less than the activity thresholds for active but >0), to 3.29 for those who were inactive.[7] After adjustment for other risk factors, the risk for active adults was 0.66 (95% CI, 0.58–0.75) and 0.77 (95% CI, 0.67–0.87) for somewhat active adults compared with inactive adults.[7]

Diet

One of the standard methods for measuring diet is the Alternative Healthy Eating Index (AHEI), a composite measure of dietary quality based on foods and nutrients that consists of 11 dietary components, each scored on a 10-point scale (0 points, least healthy; 10 points, most healthy; maximal points, 110).[7,8] The 10 components (minimum vs maximum score) include vegetables (0 vs ≥5 servings/d), fruit (0 vs ≥4 servings/d), whole grains (0 vs ≥75 g/d), sugar-sweetened beverages and fruit juice (≥1 vs 0 servings/d), nuts and legumes (0 vs ≥1 serving/d), red/processed meat (≥1.5 vs 0 servings/d), trans fat (>4% vs ≤0.5% of energy/d), long-chain (n = 3) fats (eicosapentaenoic acid plus decosohexanoic acid) (0 vs 250 mg/d), polyunsaturated fatty acids (≤2% vs ≥10% of energy/d), sodium mg/d (5271 mg/d for men ≥ 3337 mg/d for women vs ≤ 1112 mg/d for women ≤ 1612 mg/d for men), alcoholic drinks (≥3.5 vs 0.5–2 drinks/d). Among participants in the Nurse's Health study and The Health Professionals Follow-up Study who were free of chronic disease at baseline, those in the lowest quintile of diet scores were more likely to develop coronary artery disease or diabetes than those in the highest quintile.[8] Among participants in the Women's Health Study, women with an AHEI in the highest dietary quintile (score>58) had an incidence of heart failure of 17 per 10,000 person-years, which was half the incidence (34 per 10,000 person-years) seen in those in the lowest dietary quintile (AHEI score <35).[9] In multivariate analysis, women in the highest AHEI quintile had a hazard ratio of 0.70 (95% CI, 0.59, 0.82) for incident heart failure compared with those in the lowest quintile.[9]

Healthy Lifestyle

A recent study from the Women's Health Initiative examined what the investigators considered to be a healthy lifestyle and its impact on the development of heart failure.[7] They included diet, activity, smoking, and obesity. It can be argued that obesity is an outcome (with a strong genetic component) and should not be grouped with diet, activity, and smoking, which are processes. Putting these limitations aside, the data suggest that people who are able to maintain a healthy lifestyle have a significantly lower risk of heart failure than those who are unable to maintain those lifestyles.[7]

ARE RISK FACTORS FOR HEART FAILURE IMPROVING?

Trends in risk factor prevalence up to 2008 suggest that no reduction in heart failure should be expected, because the overall risk factor profile for the US population is not improving (**Fig. 6**).[10] Smoking is in decline, but hypertension, diet, and physical activity are stable and diabetes and obesity are increasing. Thus, additional targets are needed to prevent additional cases of heart failure. Even when a clear association between the risk factor and the development of heart failure has been shown, treatment of the risk factor may not result in a decrease in heart failure. Thus, clinical trials of treatment are needed to show that heart failure is reduced by treatment.

VASCULAR DISEASE

The Heart Outcomes Prevention Evaluation (HOPE) trial enrolled 9297 patients at least 55 years of age without heart failure, but with a history of coronary artery disease, stroke, peripheral vascular disease, or diabetes plus an additional cardiovascular risk factor (hypertension, increased total cholesterol level, low high-density lipoprotein cholesterol level, cigarette smoking, or documented microalbuminuria).[11] Patients randomized to 10 mg of ramipril had lower rates of heart failure over a mean 4.5 years: 9.0% versus 11.5% for placebo (relative risk, 0.77; P<.0001). The effect of ramipril was similar for subjects with (relative risk, 0.87) and without an interim myocardial infarction (relative risk, 0.78). Ramipril was more effective for subjects with systolic blood pressure greater than the median (relative risk, 0.67) compared with those with systolic blood pressure less than the median (relative risk, 0.91; P = .02 for interaction).

POTENTIAL FOR SCREENING TO PREVENT HEART FAILURE

Several conditions must be met if screening is to be successful in preventing heart failure. First there must be a preclinical phase that lasts long enough to be detected while the patient is asymptomatic, which is the case for hypertension, and there are already guidelines recommending periodic determination of blood pressure.[12] Another target for screening to prevent heart failure is asymptomatic structural heart disease (eg, left ventricular systolic dysfunction [LVSD]). The second screening condition that must be met is that treatment during the asymptomatic phase reduces the incidence of heart failure. Again, this has been shown for hypertension and for patients with ischemic heart disease. There are studies indicating that treating asymptomatic LVSD with ACE inhibitors and β-blockers prevents heart failure (discussed later). In addition, the benefits of treatment must outweigh the cost of screening. If all these conditions are met, then screening is worth pursuing.

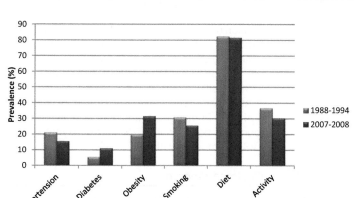

Fig. 6. Trends in risk factor prevalence to 2008. (*Data from* Huffman MD, Capewell S, Ning H, et al. Cardiovascular health behavior and health factor changes (1988–2008) and projections to 2020: results from the National Health and Nutrition Examination Surveys. Circulation 2012;125:2595–602.)

TREATABLE PRECLINICAL HEART DISEASE (STAGE B)

Several studies have examined the benefit of treating asymptomatic LVSD. Although there is evidence that treating hypertension reduces the risk of heart failure, there are few data to conclude that patients with left ventricular hypertrophy should be treated differently. However, there are insufficient data to indicate that treating asymptomatic diastolic dysfunction or most valve disease will improve outcome.

Angiotensin-converting Enzyme Inhibitors

The Studies of Left Ventricular Dysfunction (SOLVD) prevention trial showed that treatment of asymptomatic LVSD with enalapril reduced the incidence of heart failure and improved survival compared with subjects treated with placebo.[13] The median length of time to the development of heart failure was 8.3 months in the placebo group compared with 22.3 months for the enalapril group. Overall, 39% of patients in the placebo group developed heart failure compared with 30% of those in the enalapril group. Enalapril was effective in preventing cardiac deaths (odds ratio, 0.86 [0.79–0.93]) as well as total mortality (odds ratio, 0.84 [0.77–0.93]). This risk reduction led to an extension of life expectancy by 9·2 months with enalapril.

β-Blockers

A post-hoc analysis of the SOLVD prevention trial suggested that β-blockers also reduce heart failure in patients with asymptomatic LVSD. Among SOLVD trial participants, 3208 were not taking a β-blocker and 1015 were taking the drug.[14] β-Blockers reduced the risk of development of heart failure or death for patients taking enalapril (odds ratio, 0.64 [0.49–0.83]), and those taking placebo (odds ratio, 0.89 [0.72–1.12]). Post–myocardial infarction trials have also found a benefit of treating patients with β-blockers who have asymptomatic LVSD.[15,16]

The findings from these studies have led to guideline recommendations that ACE inhibitors and β-blockers be used for patients identified with asymptomatic LVSD. However, there are no guidelines for screening to detect asymptomatic LVSD.

TEAM-BASED APPROACH TO TREATMENT OF ASYMPTOMATIC LEFT VENTRICULAR SYSTOLIC DYSFUNCTION

A team-based approach to treatment of asymptomatic LVSD can work well with the availability of electronic medical records and a population approach to health. Echocardiographic or other imaging databases can be merged with outpatient and inpatient administrative and problem list data to find patients with LVSD and no prior diagnosis of heart failure. Such a list can be merged with pharmacy data to exclude patients already treated with ACE inhibitors and β-blockers. Any allergies or other intolerances of these medications can be identified. A team member can then review the list to confirm candidacy for treatment. Selected patients can then be called in for a visit with a team pharmacist to discuss treatment and begin dose titration if needed. Once the titration is complete the patient can return to the regular appointment schedule.

SCREENING TESTS

In order for screening to be successful there must be tests available with acceptable accuracy. The 2 most widely evaluated tests are B-type natriuretic peptide (BNP) and N-terminal pro-BNP (NT-proBNP).

B-type Natriuretic Peptide and N-terminal Pro–B-type Natriuretic Peptide

Vasan and colleagues[17] examined the potential of BNP to screen for LVSD in the Framingham Heart Study population. Among 3177 men with no prior diagnosis of heart failure, 70 (2.2%) had moderate to severe LVSD. The area under the receiver operating curve (AUC) for use of BNP to detect LVSD was 0.79 for men and 0.85 for women. The investigators examined a highly specific BNP screening threshold of 51 pg/mL (specificity 95%, sensitivity 33%). A systematic review of BNP to detect LVSD found similar test characteristics for BNP screening.[18] The investigators of these studies concluded that the performance of BNP to detect LVSD was too poor to justify screening.[17,18]

More recent studies have evaluated both BNP and NT-proBNP in the general population of Olmsted County, Minnesota.[19] Of 1869 patients screened, 37 had reduced left ventricular ejection fraction (LVEF) (≤40%; Table 1). The AUC for BNP (cutoff, 66 pg/mL) was 0.89, with a sensitivity and specificity of 81%. The AUC for NT-proBNP (cutoff, 228 pg/mL) was slightly higher at 0.94, with 87% sensitivity and 86% specificity.

Atrial natriuretic peptide has been evaluated in both the Framingham and UK populations and found to be inferior in detecting asymptomatic LVSD compared with BNP.[17,20,21]

Electrocardiogram

The electrocardiogram (ECG) was compared with BNP in a population without known heart failure

Table 1
Studies of BNP and NT-proBNP ability to detect asymptomatic left ventricular dysfunction

Year	Population	LVSD Definition (%)	Prevalence	Test	Threshold	Sensitivity	Specificity
2002	Framingham[17]	<40	2.2% (70 of 3177)	BNP	51 pg/ml	33%	95%
2003	General Population, United Kingdom[21]	≤35	1.6% (17 of 1058)	BNP	19 pg/ml	100%	44%
2003	General Population, United Kingdom[21]	≤35	1.6% (17 of 1058)	NT-proBNP	38 pg/ml	100%	47%
2004	Age ≥45 y, no heart failure, Olmsted County, MN[30]	≤40	1.1% (22 of 2042)	BNP	55 pg/ml	90%	76%
2004	Age >65 y, no heart failure, Olmsted County, MN[30]	≤40	2% (9 of 431)	BNP	75 pg/ml	80%	72%
2006	General male population Copenhagen, Denmark[31]	≤40	0.4% (14 of 3497; all patients)	NT-proBNP	17 pg/ml	100%	56%
2006	General female population, Copenhagen, Denmark[31]	≤40			30 pg/ml	100%	66%
2006	Olmsted County, MN[19]	≤50	6.2% (115 of 1869)	NT-proBNP	129 pg/ml	74%	74%
2006	Olmsted County, MN[19]	≤40	2.0% (37 of 1869)	NT-proBNP	228 pg/ml	86%	86%
2013	Age 65–84[32]	≤50	1.5% (22 of 1452)	NT-proBNP	278 pg/ml	64%	89%
2013	High risk[32]	≤50	1.4% (6 of 445)	NT-proBNP	278 pg/ml	100%	81%

Data from Refs.[17,19,21,30–32]

by Ng and colleagues.[21] ECG was inferior to BNP for screening purposes. Using any abnormality on ECG as a positive result had an 88% sensitivity for LVEF of less than 40% but only a 3% positive predictive value.

COST-EFFECTIVENESS MODELS OF SCREENING FOR PRECLINICAL DISEASE TO PREVENT HEART FAILURE

Several decision models have been constructed to estimate the costs and benefits of screening for reduced LVEF.[22,23] These studies modeled the long-term cost and outcome of screening a population for LVSD. In one study[22] that used BNP performance data from Framingham,[17] screening 1000 asymptomatic patients with BNP followed by echocardiography in those with an abnormal test increased the lifetime cost of care ($176,000 for men, $101,000 for women) and improved outcome (7.9 quality-adjusted life-years [QALYs] for men, 1.3 QALYs for women), resulting in a cost per QALY of $22,000 for men and $78,000 for women. For populations with a prevalence of depressed ejection fraction of at least 1%, screening with BNP followed by echocardiography increased outcome at a cost of less than $50,000 per QALY gained. The ACC/AHA consider this to be a good value in that it is within 1 gross domestic product per capita for the United States (approximately $50,000).[24] Those technologies that cost more than 3 times the gross domestic product per capita ($150,000) per year of life gained are considered a poor value.

COST-EFFECTIVENESS OF SCREENING TO PREVENT HEART FAILURE IN SPECIAL POPULATIONS: CHILDHOOD CANCER SURVIVORS

An increased risk of heart failure is known following treatment of many cancers. Given the long time delay (often decades) between anticancer treatment and the development of heart failure, the prevention of heart failure is a health care opportunity for survivors of childhood cancer. It is estimated that heart failure develops in 3% to 6% of all childhood cancer survivors, with a lifetime risk of 23% of developing, and 11% of dying from, heart failure.[25,26]

Optimal Screening Strategy for Childhood Cancer

Current guidelines recommend annual echocardiography for patients who have received 300 mg/m² of doxorubicin or equivalent.[27] The cost-effectiveness of this approach was recently modeled by Yeh and colleagues.[28] They compared annual echocardiography with echocardiograms every 2, 5, or 10 years and with no cardiac assessment. They assumed that treatment with ACE inhibitors and β-blockers reduced the risk of developing heart failure by 34% (relative risk, 0.64). Using these assumptions, imaging every 10 years improved survival at an increased cost per life-year gained of 116,000 compared with no imaging. More frequent imaging led to values of more than $150,000/life-year gained and is viewed as a poor value. Their conclusion is that imaging can be effective but is only cost-effective if done more often than every 5 years.

TEAM-BASED IMPLEMENTATION OF SCREENING TO PREVENT HEART FAILURE
STOP-HF Trial

A large randomized controlled trial (STOP-HF) of screening for asymptomatic LVEF was recently published.[29] The study included 1374 participants from 2005 to 2009 who were aged 40 years or older and had no heart failure but 1 or more of the following conditions putting them at risk for heart failure: hypertension, hypercholesterolemia, obesity, vascular disease, diabetes mellitus, arrhythmias, or moderate to severe valvular heart disease. Patients were randomized to BNP screening or usual care. BNP testing occurred annually and patients with a BNP level greater than or equal to 50 pg/mL underwent echocardiography followed by collaborative care between their primary care physician and cardiology. Primary outcomes were diagnosis of reduced LVEF or significant diastolic dysfunction. Secondary end points included emergency hospitalization for heart failure, myocardial infarction, arrhythmia, transient ischemic attack, stroke, peripheral thrombus, or pulmonary embolus. During a mean 4.2 years of follow-up, a BNP level of 50 pg/mL or more was found in 263 (42%) in the screening group, and left ventricular dysfunction was found in 58 (8.7%) of 677 in the control group and 37 (5.3%) of 697 in the screening group (P = .003). Heart failure leading to hospitalization occurred in 14 (2.1%) of 677 in the control group and 7 (1.0%) of 697 in the screening group.

Patients in the screening group had more tests, including electrocardiograms, cardiac imaging, stress testing, and ambulatory blood pressure testing, but fewer chest radiographs than those in the control group. During follow-up, intervention group patients received significantly more angiotensin receptor blocker medication and a nonsignificant increase in ACE inhibitor and mineralocorticoid antagonist medication.

Cardiovascular events were reduced from 40.4 per 1000 patient-years in the control group to 22.3 per 1000 patient-years in the intervention group (incidence rate ratio, 0.60; P = .002). Thus, the increase in cost caused by screening, follow-up testing, and specialist care is at least partially offset by fewer hospitalizations. However, a formal cost-effectiveness analysis is needed to determine whether the patient benefits are worth the increase in cost of care.

Implementing Screening in the Community to Prevent Heart Failure

The STOP-HF trial suggests how screening can be implemented by teams in the community. For large medical groups that are capitated for a patient population, clinicians with expertise in heart failure can work with their primary colleagues to define a screening policy similar to that used in the STOP-HF trial. If the group is paid by fee-for-service, it first needs to determine that screening tests will be reimbursed. A protocol should be created that defines follow-up care for patients who screen positive. For example, if a BNP threshold is used, will all patients undergo echocardiography, be referred to a specialist, or undergo some other evaluation? Attention should be given to optimizing risk factor reduction and preventive treatment with ACE inhibitors/angiotensin receptor blockers and β-blockers if LSVD is present, which is ideally done through a collaboration of primary and cardiology care. Although the data from STOP-HF suggest that heart failure can be prevented by screening at-risk patients followed by collaboration between primary care and cardiology, additional studies are needed to confirm the findings in other populations, establish the cost-effectiveness of screening, and determine optimal care for patients who screen positive. Whatever strategy is ultimately found to be useful in preventing heart failure, the implementation will require a team-based approach to population health.

REFERENCES

1. Heidenreich PA, Albert NM, Allen LA, et al. Forecasting the impact of heart failure in the United States: a policy statement from the American Heart Association. Circ Heart Fail 2013;6:606–19.
2. Hunt SA, Abraham WT, Chin MH, et al. 2009 focused update incorporated into the ACC/AHA 2005 guidelines for the diagnosis and management of heart failure in adults: a report of the American College of Cardiology Foundation/American Heart Association Task Force on Practice Guidelines: developed in collaboration with the International Society for Heart and Lung Transplantation. Circulation 2009;119: e391–479.
3. Dunlay SM, Weston SA, Jacobsen SJ, et al. Risk factors for heart failure: a population-based case-control study. Am J Med 2009;122:1023–8.
4. He J, Ogden LG, Bazzano LA, et al. Risk factors for congestive heart failure in US men and women: NHANES I epidemiologic follow-up study. Arch Intern Med 2001;161:996–1002.
5. Sciarretta S, Palano F, Tocci G, et al. Antihypertensive treatment and development of heart failure in hypertension: a bayesian network meta-analysis of studies in patients with hypertension and high cardiovascular risk. Arch Intern Med 2011;171:384–94.
6. Bangalore S, Wild D, Parkar S, et al. Beta-blockers for primary prevention of heart failure in patients with hypertension insights from a meta-analysis. J Am Coll Cardiol 2008;52:1062–72.
7. Agha G, Loucks EB, Tinker LF, et al. Healthy lifestyle and decreasing risk of heart failure in women: the Women's Health Initiative Observational Study. J Am Coll Cardiol 2014;64:1777–85.
8. Chiuve SE, Fung TT, Rimm EB, et al. Alternative dietary indices both strongly predict risk of chronic disease. J Nutr 2012;142:1009–18.
9. Belin RJ, Greenland P, Allison M, et al. Diet quality and the risk of cardiovascular disease: the Women's Health Initiative (WHI). Am J Clin Nutr 2011;94:49–57.
10. Huffman MD, Capewell S, Ning H, et al. Cardiovascular health behavior and health factor changes (1988–2008) and projections to 2020: results from the National Health and Nutrition Examination Surveys. Circulation 2012;125:2595–602.
11. Arnold JM, Yusuf S, Young J, et al. Prevention of heart failure in patients in the Heart Outcomes Prevention Evaluation (HOPE) study. Circulation 2003; 107:1284–90.
12. van Buuren S, Boshuizen HC, Reijneveld SA. Toward targeted hypertension screening guidelines. Med Decis Making 2006;26:145–53.
13. Effect of enalapril on mortality and the development of heart failure in asymptomatic patients with reduced left ventricular ejection fractions. The SOLVD Investigators. N Engl J Med 1992;327:685–91.
14. Exner DV, Dries DL, Waclawiw MA, et al. Beta-adrenergic blocking agent use and mortality in patients with asymptomatic and symptomatic left ventricular systolic dysfunction: a post hoc analysis of the studies of left ventricular dysfunction. J Am Coll Cardiol 1999;33:916–23.
15. Dargie HJ. Effect of carvedilol on outcome after myocardial infarction in patients with left-ventricular dysfunction: the CAPRICORN randomised trial. Lancet 2001;357:1385–90.
16. Pfeffer MA, Braunwald E, Moye LA, et al. Effect of captopril on mortality and morbidity in patients with left ventricular dysfunction after myocardial infarction. Results of the Survival and Ventricular Enlargement Trial. The SAVE Investigators. N Engl J Med 1992;327:669–77.
17. Vasan RS, Benjamin EJ, Larson MG, et al. Plasma natriuretic peptides for community screening for left ventricular hypertrophy and systolic dysfunction: the Framingham Heart Study. JAMA 2002;288:1252–9.
18. Wang TJ, Levy D, Benjamin EJ, et al. The epidemiology of "asymptomatic" left ventricular systolic dysfunction: implications for screening. Ann Intern Med 2003;138:907–16.
19. Costello-Boerrigter LC, Boerrigter G, Redfield MM, et al. Amino-terminal pro-b-type natriuretic peptide and b-type natriuretic peptide in the general community: determinants and detection of left ventricular dysfunction. J Am Coll Cardiol 2006; 47:345–53.
20. McDonagh TA, Robb SD, Murdoch DR, et al. Biochemical detection of left-ventricular systolic dysfunction. Lancet 1998;351:9–13.
21. Ng LL, Loke I, Davies JE, et al. Identification of previously undiagnosed left ventricular systolic dysfunction: community screening using natriuretic peptides and electrocardiography. Eur J Heart Fail 2003;5:775–82.
22. Heidenreich PA, Gubens MA, Fonarow GC, et al. Cost-effectiveness of screening with b-type natriuretic peptide to identify patients with reduced left ventricular ejection fraction. J Am Coll Cardiol 2004;43:1019–26.

23. Nielsen OW, McDonagh TA, Robb SD, et al. Retrospective analysis of the cost-effectiveness of using plasma brain natriuretic peptide in screening for left ventricular systolic dysfunction in the general population. J Am Coll Cardiol 2003;41:113–20.

24. Anderson JL, Heidenreich PA, Barnett PG, et al. ACC/AHA statement on cost/value methodology in clinical practice guidelines and performance measures: a report of the American College of Cardiology/American Heart Association Task Force on Performance Measures and Task Force on Practice Guidelines. Circulation 2014;129:2329–45.

25. Mulrooney DA, Yeazel MW, Kawashima T, et al. Cardiac outcomes in a cohort of adult survivors of childhood and adolescent cancer: retrospective analysis of the childhood cancer survivor study cohort. BMJ 2009;339:b4606.

26. van der Pal HJ, van Dalen EC, van Delden E, et al. High risk of symptomatic cardiac events in childhood cancer survivors. J Clin Oncol 2012;30:1429–37.

27. Shankar SM, Marina N, Hudson MM, et al. Monitoring for cardiovascular disease in survivors of childhood cancer: report from the Cardiovascular Disease Task Force of the Children's Oncology Group. Pediatrics 2008;121:e387–96.

28. Yeh JM, Nohria A, Diller L. Routine echocardiography screening for asymptomatic left ventricular dysfunction in childhood cancer survivors: a model-based estimation of the clinical and economic effects. Ann Intern Med 2014;160:661–71.

29. Ledwidge M, Gallagher J, Conlon C, et al. Natriuretic peptide-based screening and collaborative care for heart failure: the STOP-HF randomized trial. JAMA 2013;310:66–74.

30. Redfield MM, Rodeheffer RJ, Jacobsen SJ, et al. Plasma brain natriuretic peptide to detect preclinical ventricular systolic or diastolic dysfunction: a community-based study. Circulation 2004;109: 3176–81.

31. Goetze JP, Mogelvang R, Maage L, et al. Plasma pro-b-type natriuretic peptide in the general population: screening for left ventricular hypertrophy and systolic dysfunction. Eur Heart J 2006;27:3004–10.

32. Mureddu GF, Tarantini L, Agabiti N, et al. Evaluation of different strategies for identifying asymptomatic left ventricular dysfunction and pre-clinical (stage B) heart failure in the elderly. Results from 'PREDICTOR', a population based-study in central Italy. Eur J Heart Fail 2013;15:1102–12.

Team-based Care for Patients Hospitalized with Heart Failure

Paul M. Larsen, MD[a], John R. Teerlink, MD, FACC, FAHA, FESC, FRCP[b],*

KEYWORDS

- Acute heart failure • Team-based • Hospitalized • Interdisciplinary • Therapeutics

KEY POINTS

- Heart failure (HF) is a major cause of morbidity and mortality in the United States, and will continue to receive increasing scrutiny in the era of cost-effective and patient-centered medicine.
- Most of the literature on team-based care of patients with HF comes from non-MD providers on the team.
- Team-based care in HF can reduce mortality, hospitalizations, length of stay, and readmissions.

INTRODUCTION

Heart failure (HF) is a major cause of admission in the United States. It is listed as the primary diagnosis in more than 1 million hospitalizations annually, and as a secondary diagnosis in 3 million hospitalizations, making HF the leading cause of hospitalization in patients older than 65.[1] Hospitalization for HF is a growing issue in the public health sector,[2] as these admissions have led to an overwhelming economic burden. More than $15.0 billion of the $30.7 billion that is spent in the United States on HF-related care is spent in the impatient setting. In contrast, this is greater than 800% more than the cost of physician office visits for HF ($1.8 billion, in 2013).[1] In the United States, the lifetime risk of developing HF is approximately 20% for those older than 40. More than 850,000 new cases are diagnosed each year,[1] and the incidence increases with age, ranging from approximately 2% in Americans aged 65 to 69, to more than 8% in those older than 85.[3] Approximately 5.7 million people in the United States have HF, and the prevalence continues to increase.

Against this backdrop, many of the largest stakeholders began to issue guidelines in hopes of improving HF care. The Centers for Medicare and Medicaid Services has adopted performance measures set out by the American College of Cardiology Foundation (ACCF) and the American Heart Association (AHA).[4] At the same time, the most recent ACCF/AHA guidelines published in 2013 have added a section dedicated to the care of patients hospitalized with HF.[5]

Despite these efforts, postdischarge outcomes after admissions for HF remain high. Thirty-day readmission,[6] 1-year postdischarge mortality,[7] and 5-year mortality rates[8] have remained relatively unchanged at 25%, 30%, and 50%, respectively. HF remains a factor in more than 10% of deaths in the United States, and approximately 7% of all cardiovascular deaths can be directly attributed to HF.[1]

Conflicts of Interest: None.
a Division of Internal Medicine, School of Medicine, University of California San Francisco, 505 Parnassus Avenue, San Francisco, CA 94143, USA; b Section of Cardiology, San Francisco Veterans Affairs Medical Center, School of Medicine, University of California San Francisco, Cardiology 111C, Building 203/Room 2A49, 4150 Clement Street, San Francisco, CA 94121-1545, USA
* Corresponding author.
E-mail address: john.teerlink@ucsf.edu

In the face of this incredible morbidity and mortality, there are relatively few studies that address multidisciplinary or team-based care for patients with HF. Even fewer are set in the inpatient hospital setting. However, there is a small but growing body of literature that demonstrates improved outcomes with a team-based inpatient model. This review provides a guide to team-based care for patients hospitalized with HF.

ASSEMBLING A TEAM

To provide effective team-based care, defining the members of the team is a logical starting point. For an inpatient HF program, a team will be needed to drive process improvement and should involve all of the stakeholders in the program.[9] The team should be interdisciplinary (**Fig. 1**), and may vary from institution to institution. If launching a new HF program, it may be easier to start with a smaller team and then expand later. The roles of some of the different team members involved in the care of the HF patient in the hospital include the following:

Administration

Before the patient sets foot in the hospital, team-based HF treatment is doomed to fail without support of the hospital administration. Building an HF team requires dedicated staff and financial resources. In an ideal setting, the HF team will have an administrator who can support the program at executive levels, providing the necessary funds to establish and maintain the team.

Emergency Department

Although HF is predominantly an outpatient, chronic condition, almost all patients with HF will experience an exacerbation with symptoms serious enough to necessitate a visit to the emergency department (ED).[10] Emergency medicine physicians are an essential part of the HF team, as they are the first to initiate processes of care, from diagnosis to therapies to disposition. The recognition of their importance in early management of these patients has led to a recent consensus document outlining this crucial role.[11]

Additionally, with the increasing use of observation units, ED personnel may become the sole care providers for a proportion of urgent HF care.[12]

Cardiologist

A cardiologist provides medical knowledge and experience not only for the management of HF and its multiple underlying causes, but also for the interpretation of diagnostics and selection of therapies. During the initial phase of the construction of an HF team, a physician leader can coordinate decisions about workflow, processes, and protocols, as well as fight resistance to the program.[9] The cardiologist is uniquely qualified for this role and studies from the past 2 decades have shown that cardiologists are best suited to guide the care of hospitalized patients with HF and have better clinical outcomes.[13]

Hospitalist

The number of hospitalists in the United States has risen dramatically in the past 20 years. The American Hospital Association and Society of Hospital Medicine estimate that there were approximately 30,000 hospitalists in the United States in 2010.[14] Because of the specialty's relative newness, there are few data in the published literature about the demographics of these practicing hospitalists. However, with the profession's rapid growth, it is reasonable to assume that they will be involved in the day-to-day management of patients with HF. Obtaining their investment in the program is crucial to coordinate care and implement quality improvement initiatives.

Nurses, Nurse Practitioners, and Physician Assistants

Multiple nurse roles are important in the care of the patient with HF. In daily care, they administer medications, provide patient education, assess for improvement or worsening of symptoms, and monitor the patient's response to therapies.[15] Nurses also are expanding their scope of practice as new opportunities for direct care evolve. The central role for nurses in the care of these patients makes them ideal coleaders for the planning,

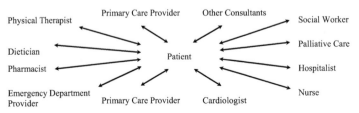

Fig. 1. A multidisciplinary HF team.

development, and activities of the HF team. Physician assistants and nurse practitioners on HF teams also have been shown to be effective and can fulfill these roles.[16]

Dietician

The diet of the patient with HF is of critical importance. Although a low-sodium diet and possibly fluid restriction may be obvious interventions, patients with HF can require complex nutritional assessments because of other comorbidities, such as diabetes, atrial fibrillation, and hyperlipidemia.[17] A dietician can provide dietary educational materials, support patients with HF in outreach or group events, and counsel individual patients with HF, as an invaluable part of the HF team.

One study found that patient education focused on sodium intake by a registered dietician improved patients' knowledge of dietary sodium intake. Awareness of the sodium restriction guideline increased threefold after education by the dietician, from 14% to 42%. The proportion of subjects who achieved a perfect sodium knowledge score was 8% at baseline and 26% at follow-up.[18]

Physical and Occupational Therapists

Patients with HF suffer from physical limitations because of reduced flexibility, conditioning, and exercise capacity. These patients are often unable to perform normal daily activities or must complete these tasks at a reduced rate. In the hospitalized patient, lengthy immobilization can lead to further debilitation. Although much of the data exists in the outpatient setting, trials have shown physical therapy to be safe, easily accepted by patients, and effective in improving global perception of symptoms and functional status.[19] Patient education about activity recommendations and strategies for dealing with deficiencies in activities of daily living can lead to lasting benefits after discharge. Occupational therapists also contribute to the transition plan by performing a safety assessment and recommending an appropriate level of care after discharge based on a patient's functional ability.

Pharmacist

Patient comorbidities, drug-drug interactions, and insurance restrictions on medications are just a few of the many factors that establish the pharmacist as a key member of the HF team. These professionals can assist greatly with the transition from outpatient medications to inpatient therapies, reconciling the complex and dynamic regimens, while ultimately preparing for discharge. Clinical

pharmacists can improve patient knowledge and medication adherence through education during an inpatient stay. In collaboration with the rest of the team, pharmacists can help ensure that evidence-based medications are initiated and drug toxicities are monitored. Inpatient studies have demonstrated that predischarge initiation of life-saving HF therapies, such as beta-blockers, in patients hospitalized for HF improved their use at 60 days without increasing side effects or length of stay.[20] Another study showed that involving a clinical pharmacist in the outpatient setting as a member of the HF team significantly increased the dose of angiotensin converting enzyme (ACE) inhibitors prescribed to patients. These patients also experienced lower all-cause mortality and HF event rates.[21]

Social Worker/Case Manager

Social workers are frequently involved in identifying various needs of patients during hospitalizations for HF. In many hospitals, they also are responsible for arranging discharge plans. The suggestion that 30-day rehospitalization rates may be greatly influenced by nonmedical, socioeconomic, and environmental factors has reinforced the important role these case managers may play. They are knowledgeable about community resources and help patients secure additional services, such as transportation or in-home nursing after discharge, and also have been shown to improve clinical outcomes.[22]

Palliative Care

In a disease process with 50% 5-year mortality, palliative care should be involved early in the HF team process for many patients in combination with curative therapy. Hospitals without access to palliative care specialists should still engage patients in goals-of-care discussions early in the disease process to allow patients and their families time to consider these important decisions.[23,24] This critical component of HF care is discussed in further detail later in this issue.

Nonclinical Staff

Nonclinical staff can play a critical role in meeting performance improvement initiatives of an HF program. Various departments, such as clinical documentation information, coding, and information services, can all aid the HF team by collecting, analyzing, and reporting HF data. They also can work to help improve the HF team workflow by creating admission order sets, discharge instructions, and clinical alerts.

Outpatient Providers

Even in the inpatient setting, collaboration with the primary care provider (PCP) must be included. By including the PCP in the HF team, better coordination of care can lead to protocols to attempt to bridge the gap between inpatient and outpatient medicine.[9] Although diagnosis and treatment by a cardiologist in the impatient setting is common, most of these patients will visit their PCP far more frequently than they visit their cardiologist. After the initial diagnosis, the PCPs play a crucial role in the implementation of evidence-based treatment and subsequent follow-up.[25] In a recent retrospective study of more than 12,000 patients treated and discharged from the ED for HF, the rate of death or all-cause hospitalization at 6 months was 11% lower in those who saw a familiar physician in the first month versus those with no outpatient visits, and 15% lower than those with visits only with unfamiliar physicians.[26]

Other Consultants

In a complex patient population with multiple co-morbidities, collaboration with noncardiology specialists is critical for early recognition and treatment of these conditions. Nephrologists, interventional cardiologists, and cardiothoracic surgeons are just a few of the many different providers who can provide additional benefit to the HF team.

IDENTIFYING PATIENTS WITH HEART FAILURE IN THE HOSPITAL

To treat patients with HF, we must first identify who has HF, and to identify HF, we must define HF. HF is not a singular disease process, but rather a complex clinical syndrome that arises from structural or functional impairment of ventricular filling or ejection of blood. The current ACCF/AHA guidelines further describe HF with preserved or reduced ejection fraction as HFpEF and HFrEF, respectively.[5] Once patients are diagnosed with HF, they need to be effectively referred to the HF team. Although this may seem both simple and self-evident, "finding" patients with HF in the hospital can be challenging. Notifications to the HF team through the ED can be through direct communication, which is dependent on the individual emergency physician provider and consequently highly variable, or through more automated processes linked to admitting diagnoses or diagnostic studies (eg, N-terminal of the prohormone brain natriuretic peptide [NT-proBNP]/BNP, echocardiogram results). Early identification of patients with HF is a priority, as it allows for earlier intervention and patient education.[27] Previously reported and emerging data support the hypothesis that acute HF is an event with early end-organ dysfunction and damage that can be treated by early initiation of therapy,[28–30] reinforcing the importance of early identification of these patients.

There is no widely accepted nomenclature for HF syndromes requiring hospitalization. Patients are often described as having "acute HF," "acute HF syndromes," or "acute (ly) decompensated HF" in various literature and in daily conversation. "Acute HF" may currently have the widest acceptance, but it still has limitations because it does not differentiate between an initial presentation of HF from a worsening of previously stable chronic HF.[5]

HF registries can provide some data as to who may require hospitalization.[31] Patients are typically older, of either sex, and often have hypertension, chronic kidney disease, hyponatremia, hematologic abnormalities, and chronic obstructive pulmonary disease (COPD). Interestingly, a relatively equal percentage of patients with acute HF have HFpEF compared with HFrEF.[32] However, the patients with HFpEF are older, less likely male, more likely to have hypertension, and have less coronary artery disease. The overall morbidity and mortality for both groups is high.

TEAM-BASED CARE THROUGHOUT THE HOSPITAL COURSE

The Emergency Department

The history

Whether making a new diagnosis of HF or encountering a patient with a long-standing HF history, the first step is to identify a patient with HF. Starting in the ED, prompt documentation of HF allows for earlier mobilization of the HF team (**Table 1**). Patients with a history of HF are the most readily diagnosed and identified; among almost 12 million Medicare beneficiaries discharged from a hospitalization, 27% of patients discharged from an index hospitalization for HF were rehospitalized within 30 days, 37% of whom were admitted for HF.[33] Despite advances in imaging and laboratory testing, the history and physical examination remain central to diagnosing and assessing patients with HF. Patients with a history of myocardial infarction, valvular disease, or severe hypertension also merit particular attention. HF should be considered as a possibility in any patient with decreased exercise tolerance, although this is a very nonspecific finding. The clinical symptoms and signs of elevated filling pressure, such as orthopnea, edema, and jugular venous distension, are more specific but typically occur later in the disease process.

Table 1
Team members' roles on the patient's path through the hospitalization

Nonclinical Staff	Pharmacist	Dietician	Therapists	Palliative Care
Coding	Patient education	Patient education	Cardiac rehabilitation	Symptom management
Collecting data	Medication review	Nutrition assessment	Safety assessment	Pain control
Reviewing records	Medication monitoring	Calorie counting	Patient education	End-of-life planning
Creating order sets	Pharmacy support	—	—	Goals of care

Emergency Provider	Cardiologist	Hospitalist	Registered Nurse	Social Worker
Resuscitation	Diagnosis	Comorbidity care	Inpatient monitoring	Home care
Diagnosis	Therapeutics	Patient education	Patient education	Transportation
Symptom relief	Patient education	Inpatient monitoring	Medicine distribution	Pharmacy support
Disposition	Monitoring	—	—	Follow-up care

Orthopnea is the patient-reported symptom that has the highest sensitivity to a baseline elevated left ventricular filling pressure.[34] Often described as shortness of breath when lying down, orthopnea also may be demonstrated by a nighttime cough. Similarly, paroxysmal nocturnal dyspnea also reflects the worsening of chronic elevation in left-sided filling pressures.[35] Weight gain, new edema, or ascites are all clear signs of volume overload.

A thorough history should include questions that attempt to divine the underlying cause of both the HF and the exacerbation. A common cause, such as previous myocardial ischemia or substance abuse, can be readily identified with simple questions, although attempting to prove causation should happen later during the hospitalization. Questions around changes to diet and adherence to medications assess for both medical awareness and access to heart-healthy food and medication.

As in all patients admitted to the hospital, no history is complete without establishing the patient's wishes with regard to potential resuscitation, interventions, and goals of care. This framework will help to establish the direction that the patient's care may take in the hospital setting. Notably, the preferences of patients with HF appear to be driven by the decline in clinical status that often accompanies advanced age and comorbidities.[36,37] In addition, these data suggest that "do-not-resuscitate" status is not an independent risk factor for a patient's death in the hospital.[36]

The role of the nonclinical staff also starts as soon as the patient enters the ED. The earlier patients with HF are identified, the earlier team-based interventions can occur. Although there is no single method of identifying all of these patients, with a mix of strategies the HF team can maximize the identification of patients with HF.

Admitting diagnosis list

An admitting diagnosis list or orders can be a useful tool to identify patients with HF in the hospital. However, HF is not always diagnosed at the time of admission. Chief complaints that describe HF symptoms, like shortness of breath or edema, merit further investigation. If the diagnosis of HF is not being made on admission, an HF order set could be used to generate HF team consults. Although the effectiveness is dependent on the physician's commitment to using them, admission order sets have been shown to reduce variability and costs, and increase quality of care.[38]

Tracking laboratory tests or therapeutics

As many patients with HF are volume overloaded, tracking patients who had BNP/NT-proBNP values drawn or who were administered intravenous diuretics offers additional ways to identify patients hospitalized with HF. In limited studies, intravenous diuretic use has been shown to be both sensitive and specific in predicting a discharge diagnosis of HF.[27]

The physical examination

The oft-repeated saying "vital signs are vital for a reason" continues to have relevance in the examination of the patient with HF. Palpation of the pulse will reveal the intensity and regularity of the pulse. Pulsus alternans, if present, suggests severe left ventricular dysfunction. Blood pressure is ideally obtained in both the supine and upright positions. Hypertension as a precipitating cause, or hypotension suggesting poor cardiac output may help guide management. If orthostatic changes to heart rate or blood pressure are present, the patient may be suffering from medication effects or excess volume depletion.

The cardiac examination helps to categorize patients based on perfusion and volume status/congestion. Jugular venous distention has been shown to be a sensitive and specific marker for an elevation in pulmonary capillary wedge pressure.[39] Elevated jugular venous pressure and third heart sounds are both independently associated with worse outcomes in patients hospitalized with HFrEF.[40] A displacement in the point of maximum impulse suggests an enlarged ventricle. Murmurs may be either causative or resulting from antecedent HF.

The respiratory status, including rate, oxygen saturation, rales, and presence of any effusions, can help elucidate volume status. It is worth noting that as HF advances, rales can be absent in the setting of pulmonary congestion. Other indicators of volume overload, such as peripheral edema, hepatomegaly, or ascites, are nonspecific markers for HF. Finally, the temperature of the extremities will help inform the clinician as to whether the patient has adequate cardiac output.

Diagnostic studies

The initial evaluation of all patients presenting with possible HF should include the following:

- 12-lead electrocardiogram
- Serum electrolytes
- Serum blood urea nitrogen
- Serum creatinine
- Serum glucose
- Serum lipids
- Serum thyroid-stimulating hormone
- Serum liver function tests
- Serum BNP or NT-proBNP
- Chest radiograph

An electrocardiogram (ECG) may provide insight as to the severity or cause of HF. Sinus tachycardia may indicate the elevated sympathetic tone seen in patients with decompensated HF, although beta-blockade may attenuate this effect. Atrial rhythm abnormalities, such as atrial fibrillation, frequently occur in patients with dilated atria from long-standing HF, and may represent either the precipitant or the result of volume overload and congestion. Low voltage can suggest tamponade, severe COPD, or cardiac amyloid. The presence of deep Q-waves may indicate that myocardial ischemia is the cause of the HF. A left bundle branch block can occur from ischemic heart disease or a nonischemic cardiomyopathy. Poor R-wave progression also is seen in both ischemic and nonischemic cardiomyopathies.

Serum electrolytes, and renal and liver function can all reflect severity of disease and can therefore be useful for management. Measurement of thyroid function, hemoglobin, or serum iron studies may indicate an underlying cause of the patient's HF. In certain populations or patients with various comorbidities, serologic testing for collagen vascular diseases, amyloidosis, pheochromocytoma, drugs of abuse, or human immunodeficiency virus is reasonable.

Over the past 20 years, cardiac biomarkers have received increasing notice for their role in both diagnosing and predicting outcomes in HF. Numerous studies support the idea that BNP or NT-proBNP are useful tools to support clinical judgment in the diagnosis of decompensated HF.[41,42] BNP correlates reasonably well with NT-proBNP, and either is recommended as long as their cutoffs are not used interchangeably.[5] It is important to note that BNP or NT-proBNP elevations are not exclusively due to HF, and are associated with a variety of other causes. Still, either biomarker can be useful when attempting to establish an initial baseline as to disease severity or to prognosticate in the patient with decompensated HF.

Cardiac troponin I or T may be the most useful non-natriuretic peptide-based biomarkers currently available. Elevated levels of cardiac troponin are often found in patients with HF,[43–46] many times without any history or other evidence of myocardial ischemia, and even in the absence of coronary artery disease. In patients with HF, the presence of elevated cardiac troponin is associated with increased mortality and worse outcomes. Additionally, a persistent elevation in troponin portends a worse prognosis in acute decompensated HF.[47]

Chest radiographs can be the initial diagnostic tool that suggests the presence of HF. Rarely, it can illustrate the cause, as with a left ventricular aneurysm or some congenital heart disease. More often, fluid in the intralobular fissures, alveoli, or pulmonary interstitium all evoke pulmonary venous hypertension and therefore possibly HF. Cardiomegaly is useful if present, but is often not seen. The chest radiograph's utility is further limited when obtained with the patient supine and shot in the anterior-posterior view. A standing, posterior-anterior film is preferred if the patient can tolerate standing.

The identification of patients with HF is not the only role for the ED provider. In conjunction with the admitting providers in the hospital, they must also focus on resuscitation, symptom palliation, and an accurate disposition, ranging from discharge to admission to the intensive care unit. Therapeutics delivered in the ED and for the admitted patient overlap to a great extent, and are covered in the following inpatient section.

INPATIENT
Precipitants and Comorbidities

Almost 60% of patients have at least one clearly identifiable precipitant in an HF hospitalization.[48] Some of the most common include the following:

- Pneumonia
- Myocardial ischemia
- Arrhythmia
- Medication noncompliance
- Hypertension
- Dietary changes

Acute coronary syndrome is imperative to diagnose as a cause of new or worsening HF. Unsurprisingly, the presence of these precipitants independently increases the chance of having a poor outcome. Many of these precipitants are already being identified by ED providers. If not, or if severe, this provides the opportunity to involve hospitalists or other consultants skilled in noncardiac care. Excessive sodium intake should prompt a visit from the dietician. Medication nonadherence or use of drugs that can precipitate acute HF, such as nonsteroidal anti-inflammatory drugs, offer a vehicle for the pharmacist to provide patient education and possibly optimize the medicine regimen.

Common comorbidities in HF overlap with its precipitants. These conditions include the following:

- Atrial fibrillation
- Coronary artery disease
- Anemia
- Depression

- COPD
- Diabetes
- Hypertension
- Renal failure

All of these comorbidities influence treatment approaches and success.[31,49] Control of these comorbidities and noncardiac conditions are covered in further detail in the following articles by Drs. Whellan and Rich, elsewhere in this issue.

Echocardiography

The most useful test for the evaluation of patients at risk for HF is a comprehensive echocardiogram. An echocardiogram can provide an assessment of the following:

- Left ventricular systolic function
- Diastolic function
- Wall thickness/hypertrophy
- Ventricular volumes and dimensions
- Regional wall motion
- Atrial size
- Valvular abnormalities and flow
- Infiltration
- Pericardial disease
- Hemodynamics

An echocardiogram can reveal subclinical systolic or diastolic dysfunction and also predict future adverse events.[50] Serial evaluations of ejection fraction are not useful unless the patient has had a significant change in clinical status, or received therapy that may affect cardiac function. Echocardiography remains preferred over other imaging modalities because of its lack of radiation and widespread use and acceptance.

Diuresis

Patients with HF who are fluid overloaded need diuretic therapy. Current guidelines suggest that intravenous loop diuretics should be given at a dose equal to or higher than their chronic oral dose, and therapy should be initiated in the ED if possible.[30] Nursing is key for monitoring the following:

- Daily weights
- Vital signs
- Electrolytes, urea nitrogen, and creatinine
- Fluid inputs and outputs
- Administering thromboembolism prophylaxis.

When initial diuretic response is not adequate, options include the addition of a second diuretic or increasing the loop diuretic dosage. Either a continuous or intermittent bolus strategy is reasonable in patients who are resistant.[51]

Thiazides are known to improve diuretic responsiveness. The addition of dopamine or nesiritide to improve diuresis has not been demonstrated to be effective[52–54] and is not currently recommended.[5]

Ultrafiltration

In patients who are refractory to intravenous diuretics, ultrafiltration can be considered. In some centers, this therapy requires a nephrologist, one of the most common consultants used by an HF team. Ultrafiltration can move water and small solutes across a membrane, thereby reducing fluid overload. Ultrafiltration has not been proven superior to bolus diuretic therapy,[55] and because of higher costs and possible adverse outcomes, it remains a rescue therapy for selected patients with HF.

Previous Therapy

The most recent ACCF/AHA guidelines designate the term guideline-directed medical therapy (GDMT) to represent optimal medical therapy.[5] On admission, the patient's previous HF medications should be reviewed by the provider, as the inpatient setting provides a chance to optimize outpatient medical therapy. For most patients, HF therapy should be continued during the hospitalization.[56,57] ACE inhibitors, angiotensin receptor blockers, or mineralocorticoid receptor antagonists may be held in the setting of renal dysfunction. Stopping or decreasing beta-blockers should occur only if they were recently started or increased, or with low cardiac output. The specialized care of the patient with low cardiac output and/or cardiogenic shock, including inotropes and supportive devices, is covered in the article by Dr. Fang, elsewhere in this issue. If initiating new beta-blocker therapy, starting with a low dose when hemodynamically stable is preferred, with special caution paid to those who require inotropic support earlier in the hospitalization.

Vasodilators

In normotensive patients experiencing dyspnea, vasodilators, including intravenous nitroglycerin, sodium nitroprusside, or nesiritide, can provide symptomatic relief.[5] Nitroglycerin may reduce pulmonary congestion by venodilation and reducing preload.[58] Sodium nitroprusside mixes venodilation and arteriodilation, but is typically reserved for the advanced HF population because of potential hypotension.[59] Nesiritide reduces left ventricular filling pressure and may provide mild dyspnea relief, but has not been shown to reduce mortality or rehospitalization.[60]

Transitions of Care and Discharge

The discharge and immediate postdischarge care of the patients with HF is a critical time, and the article by Dr. Walsh, elsewhere in this issue, is devoted to this topic. The ACCF/AHA stresses that throughout the hospitalization and discharge, it is necessary to address the following:

- Initiation of GDMT
- Causes of HF
- Volume status
- Blood pressure
- Renal function
- Electrolytes
- HF education
- Important comorbidities

Assessment of the patient's needs should begin on admission, and include input from the nurses, physical and occupational therapists, dietician, and pharmacist. Interestingly, a recent report from the Tele-HF trial found that the quality of the discharge summary and its communication to the outside physician was each associated with reduced readmission rates.[61] Comprehensive discharge planning and support can reduce readmission rates and may improve health outcomes, such as survival and quality of life, and does so without increasing costs.[62]

IS TEAM-BASED CARE EFFECTIVE?

Meta-analysis suggests that multidisciplinary management for patients with HF reduces hospitalization rates up to 27%, and reduces all-cause mortality by up to 25%.[63] In the hospitalized patient, a multidisciplinary HF team has been shown to lead to the following[64–66]:

- Higher rates of ACE inhibitor use
- Higher rates of beta-blocker use
- Increased smoking counseling
- Shorter length of stay
- Decreased cost

The relatively short time spent in the hospital when compared with the outpatient setting makes the determination of the optimal inpatient team for HF difficult. Studies vary in their team composition, ranging from a cardiologist and nurse to the extensive team detailed earlier.

SUMMARY

Management of the patient hospitalized with HF presents a unique set of challenges. With a team-based approach to HF, systems can be established to enact evidence-based guidelines, ensure quality care, and prevent mistakes in the vulnerable time immediately after discharge. The HF team can improve outcomes including quality of life, rehospitalization, and survival. The HF team is composed of members in a wide variety of departments and roles, each bringing their own expertise to patient care.

HF is a complex clinical syndrome with many precipitants and comorbidities that need to be individually addressed. While hospitalized, it allows the team to optimize GDMT and educate the patient on the importance of medication adherence, diet, and exercise. As the population continues to age and hospitals come under further scrutiny with regard to cost and quality of patient care, we should anticipate the team-based care of patients with HF to continue to take a more prominent role in providing care for this high-risk group of patients.

REFERENCES

1. Mozaffarian D, Benjamin EJ, Go AS, et al. Heart disease and stroke statistics—2015 update: a report from the American Heart Association. Circulation 2014;131(4):e29–322.
2. Fang J, Mensah GA, Croft JB, et al. Heart failure-related hospitalization in the US, 1979 to 2004. J Am Coll Cardiol 2008;52:428–34.
3. Curtis LH, Whellan DJ, Hammill BG, et al. Incidence and prevalence of heart failure in elderly persons, 1994–2003. Arch Intern Med 2008;168:418–24.
4. Bonow RO, Ganiats TG, Beam CT, et al. ACCF/AHA/AMA-PCPI 2011 performance measures for adults with heart failure: a report of the American College of Cardiology Foundation/American Heart Association Task Force on Performance Measures and the American Medical Association-Physician Consortium for Performance Improvement. Circulation 2012;125:2382–401.
5. Yancy CW, Jessup M, Bozkurt B, et al. 2013 ACCF/AHA guideline for the management of heart failure: a report of the American College of Cardiology Foundation/American Heart Association Task Force on Practice Guidelines. J Am Coll Cardiol 2013;62: e147–239.
6. Ross JS, Chen J, Lin Z, et al. Recent national trends in readmission rates after heart failure hospitalization. Circ Heart Fail 2010;3:97–103.
7. Chen J, Normand SL, Wang Y, et al. National and regional trends in heart failure hospitalization and mortality rates for Medicare beneficiaries, 1998–2008. JAMA 2011;306:1669–78.
8. Roger VL, Weston SA, Redfield MM, et al. Trends in heart failure incidence and survival in a community-based population. JAMA 2004;292:344–50.
9. Rathman LD, Basso C, Fiorini D. Genesis of an inpatient heart failure program. In: Paul S, editor. Heart

failure disease management: from planning to implementation. 1st edition. Mount Laurel (NJ): American Association of Heart Failure Nurses; 2014. p. 47–64.

10. Weintraub NL, Collins SP, Pang PS, et al. Acute heart failure syndromes: emergency department presentation, treatment, and disposition: current approaches and future aims: a scientific statement from the American Heart Association. Circulation 2010;122:1975–96.

11. Collins S, Storrow AB, Albert NM, et al. Early management of patients with acute heart failure: state of the art and future directions. A consensus document from the Society for Academic Emergency Medicine/Heart Failure Society of America Acute Heart Failure Working Group. J Card Fail 2015;21: 27–43.

12. Collins SP, Pang PS, Fonarow GC, et al. Is hospital admission for heart failure really necessary? The role of the emergency department and observation unit in preventing hospitalization and rehospitalization. J Am Coll Cardiol 2013;61:121–6.

13. Jong P, Gong Y, Liu PP, et al. Care and outcomes of patients newly hospitalized for heart failure in the community treated by cardiologists compared with other specialists. Circulation 2003;108:184–91.

14. Harbuck SM, Follmer AD, Dill MJ, et al. Estimating the number and characteristics of hospitalist physicians in the United States and their possible workforce implications. Association of American Medical Colleges 2012;12(3). Available at: https://www.aamc.org/download/300620/data/aibvol12_no3-hospitalist.pdf.

15. Jaarsma T. Inter-professional team approach to patients with heart failure. Heart 2005;91:832–8.

16. Naylor MD, Brooten DA, Campbell RL, et al. Transitional care of older adults hospitalized with heart failure: a randomized, controlled trial. J Am Geriatr Soc 2004;52:675–84.

17. Jaarsma T. Health care professionals in a heart failure team. Eur J Heart Fail 2005;7:343–9.

18. Neily JB, Toto KH, Gardner EB, et al. Potential contributing factors to noncompliance with dietary sodium restriction in patients with heart failure. Am Heart J 2002;143:29–33.

19. Corvera-Tindel T, Doering LV, Woo MA, et al. Effects of a home walking exercise program on functional status and symptoms in heart failure. Am Heart J 2004;147:339–46.

20. Gattis WA, O'Connor CM, Gallup DS, et al. Predischarge initiation of carvedilol in patients hospitalized for decompensated heart failure: results of the initiation management predischarge: process for assessment of carvedilol therapy in heart failure (IMPACT-HF) trial. J Am Coll Cardiol 2004;43:1534–41.

21. Gattis WA, Hasselblad V, Whellan DJ, et al. Reduction in heart failure events by the addition of

a clinical pharmacist to the heart failure management team: results of the Pharmacist in Heart Failure Assessment Recommendation and Monitoring (PHARM) Study. Arch Intern Med 1999; 159:1939–45.

22. Rich MW, Gray DB, Beckham V, et al. Effect of a multidisciplinary intervention on medication compliance in elderly patients with congestive heart failure. Am J Med 1996;101:270–6.

23. Goodlin SJ, Hauptman PJ, Arnold R, et al. Consensus statement: palliative and supportive care in advanced heart failure. J Card Fail 2004; 10:200–9.

24. LeMond L, Camacho SA, Goodlin SJ. Palliative care and decision making in advanced heart failure. Curr Treat Options Cardiovasc Med 2015;17:359.

25. Hobbs FD. Primary care physicians: champions of or an impediment to optimal care of the patient with heart failure? Eur J Heart Fail 1999;1:11–5.

26. Sidhu RS, Youngson E, McAlister FA. Physician continuity improves outcomes for heart failure patients treated and released from the emergency department. JACC Heart Fail 2014;2:368–76.

27. Halasyamani LK, Czerwinski J, Clinard R, et al. An electronic strategy to identify hospitalized heart failure patients. J Hosp Med 2007;2:409–14.

28. Metra M, Cotter G, Davison BA, et al. Effect of serelaxin on cardiac, renal, and hepatic biomarkers in the relaxin in acute heart failure (RELAX-AHF) development program: correlation with outcomes. J Am Coll Cardiol 2013;61:196–206.

29. Teerlink JR, Cotter G, Davison BA, et al. Serelaxin, recombinant human relaxin-2, for treatment of acute heart failure (RELAX-AHF): a randomised, placebo-controlled trial. Lancet 2013;381:29–39.

30. Peacock WF 4th, Fonarow GC, Emerman CL, et al. Impact of early initiation of intravenous therapy for acute decompensated heart failure on outcomes in ADHERE. Cardiology 2007;107:44–51.

31. Adams KF Jr, Fonarow GC, Emerman CL, et al. Characteristics and outcomes of patients hospitalized for heart failure in the United States: rationale, design, and preliminary observations from the first 100,000 cases in the Acute Decompensated Heart Failure National Registry (ADHERE). Am Heart J 2005;149:209–16.

32. West R, Liang L, Fonarow GC, et al. Characterization of heart failure patients with preserved ejection fraction: a comparison between ADHERE-US registry and ADHERE-International registry. Eur J Heart Fail 2011;13:945–52.

33. Jencks SF, Williams MV, Coleman EA. Rehospitalizations among patients in the Medicare fee-for-service program. N Engl J Med 2009;360:1418–28.

34. Stevenson LW, Perloff JK. The limited reliability of physical signs for estimating hemodynamics in chronic heart failure. JAMA 1989;261:884–8.

35. Kannel WB, Belanger AJ. Epidemiology of heart failure. Am Heart J 1991;121:951–7.

36. Dunlay SM, Swetz KM, Redfield MM, et al. Resuscitation preferences in community patients with heart failure. Circ Cardiovasc Qual Outcomes 2014;7:353–9.

37. Dev S, Clare RM, Felker GM, et al. Link between decisions regarding resuscitation and preferences for quality over length of life with heart failure. Eur J Heart Fail 2012;14:45–53.

38. Ballard DJ, Ogola G, Fleming NS, et al. Impact of a standardized heart failure order set on mortality, readmission, and quality and costs of care. Int J Qual Health Care 2010;22:437–44.

39. Butman SM, Ewy GA, Standen JR, et al. Bedside cardiovascular examination in patients with severe chronic heart failure: importance of rest or inducible jugular venous distension. J Am Coll Cardiol 1993; 22:968–74.

40. Drazner MH, Rame JE, Stevenson LW, et al. Prognostic importance of elevated jugular venous pressure and a third heart sound in patients with heart failure. N Engl J Med 2001;345:574–81.

41. Maisel AS, McCord J, Nowak RM, et al. Bedside B-Type natriuretic peptide in the emergency diagnosis of heart failure with reduced or preserved ejection fraction. Results from the breathing not properly multinational study. J Am Coll Cardiol 2003;41:2010–7.

42. Mueller C, Scholer A, Laule-Kilian K, et al. Use of B-type natriuretic peptide in the evaluation and management of acute dyspnea. N Engl J Med 2004; 350:647–54.

43. Peacock WF 4th, De Marco T, Fonarow GC, et al. Cardiac troponin and outcome in acute heart failure. N Engl J Med 2008;358:2117–26.

44. O'Connor CM, Fiuzat M, Lombardi C, et al. Impact of serial troponin release on outcomes in patients with acute heart failure: analysis from the PROTECT pilot study. Circ Heart Fail 2011;4:724–32.

45. Braga JR, Tu JV, Austin PC, et al. Outcomes and care of patients with acute heart failure syndromes and cardiac troponin elevation. Circ Heart Fail 2013;6:193–202.

46. Metra M, Ponikowski P, Cotter G, et al. Effects of serelaxin in subgroups of patients with acute heart failure: results from RELAX-AHF. Eur Heart J 2013;34: 3128–36.

47. Ather S, Hira RS, Shenoy M, et al. Recurrent low-level troponin I elevation is a worse prognostic indicator than occasional injury pattern in patients hospitalized with heart failure. Int J Cardiol 2013; 166:394–8.

48. Fonarow GC, Abraham WT, Albert NM, et al. Factors identified as precipitating hospital admissions for heart failure and clinical outcomes: findings from OPTIMIZE-HF. Arch Intern Med 2008;168:847–54.

49. O'Connor CM, Stough WG, Gallup DS, et al. Demographics, clinical characteristics, and outcomes of patients hospitalized for decompensated heart failure: observations from the IMPACT-HF registry. J Card Fail 2005;11:200–5.

50. Agha SA, Kalogeropoulos AP, Shih J, et al. Echocardiography and risk prediction in advanced heart failure: incremental value over clinical markers. J Card Fail 2009;15:586–92.

51. Felker GM, Lee KL, Bull DA, et al. Diuretic strategies in patients with acute decompensated heart failure. N Engl J Med 2011;364:797–805.

52. Triposkiadis FK, Butler J, Karayannis G, et al. Efficacy and safety of high dose versus low dose furosemide with or without dopamine infusion: the dopamine in acute decompensated heart failure II (DAD-HF II) trial. Int J Cardiol 2014;172:115–21.

53. Giamouzis G, Butler J, Starling RC, et al. Impact of dopamine infusion on renal function in hospitalized heart failure patients: results of the Dopamine in Acute Decompensated Heart Failure (DAD-HF) trial. J Card Fail 2010;16:922–30.

54. Chen HH, Anstrom KJ, Givertz MM, et al. Low-dose dopamine or low-dose nesiritide in acute heart failure with renal dysfunction: the ROSE acute heart failure randomized trial. JAMA 2013;310:2533–43.

55. Bart BA, Goldsmith SR, Lee KL, et al. Ultrafiltration in decompensated heart failure with cardiorenal syndrome. N Engl J Med 2012;367:2296–304.

56. Fonarow GC, Abraham WT, Albert NM, et al. Influence of beta-blocker continuation or withdrawal on outcomes in patients hospitalized with heart failure: findings from the OPTIMIZE-HF program. J Am Coll Cardiol 2008;52:190–9.

57. Metra M, Torp-Pedersen C, Cleland JG, et al. Should beta-blocker therapy be reduced or withdrawn after an episode of decompensated heart failure? Results from COMET. Eur J Heart Fail 2007;9:901–9.

58. Cotter G, Metzkor E, Kaluski E, et al. Randomised trial of high-dose isosorbide dinitrate plus low-dose furosemide versus high-dose furosemide plus low-dose isosorbide dinitrate in severe pulmonary oedema. Lancet 1998;351:389–93.

59. Mullens W, Abrahams Z, Francis GS, et al. Sodium nitroprusside for advanced low-output heart failure. J Am Coll Cardiol 2008;52:200–7.

60. O'Connor CM, Starling RC, Hernandez AF, et al. Effect of nesiritide in patients with acute decompensated heart failure. N Engl J Med 2011;365: 32–43.

61. Al-Damluji MS, Dzara K, Hodshon B, et al. Association of discharge summary quality with readmission risk for patients hospitalized with heart failure exacerbation. Circ Cardiovasc Qual Outcomes 2015;8: 109–11.

62. Phillips CO, Wright SM, Kern DE, et al. Comprehensive discharge planning with postdischarge support for older patients with congestive heart failure: a meta-analysis. JAMA 2004;291:1358–67.

63. McAlister FA, Stewart S, Ferrua S, et al. Multidisciplinary strategies for the management of heart failure patients at high risk for admission: a systematic review of randomized trials. J Am Coll Cardiol 2004;44:810–9.

64. Costantini O, Huck K, Carlson MD, et al. Impact of a guideline-based disease management team on outcomes of hospitalized patients with congestive heart failure. Arch Intern Med 2001;161:177–82.

65. Coons JC, Fera T. Multidisciplinary team for enhancing care for patients with acute myocardial infarction or heart failure. Am J Health Syst Pharm 2007;64:1274–8.

66. Gregory D, Kimmelstiel C, Perry K, et al. Hospital cost effect of a heart failure disease management program: the Specialized Primary and Networked Care in Heart Failure (SPAN-CHF) trial. Am Heart J 2006;151:1013–8.

Team-Based Transitions of Care in Heart Failure

Judy Tingley, MPH, RN[a], Mary A. Dolansky, PhD, RN[b], Mary Norine Walsh, MD[c],*

KEYWORDS

• Heart failure • Transitions of care • Team-based care

KEY POINTS

- With the implementation of the Patient Protection and Affordable Care Act, the requisite for health care systems to build team-based transitional care programs is clear.
- The clinical course for patients with heart failure is complicated and progressive, which leads to frequent acute care hospitalization and higher mortality.
- Research and advocacy efforts need to continue to facilitate the team-based approach to transitions and improve the quality of care.

INTRODUCTION

Heart failure (HF) affects 5.1 million people in the United States, and in 2009, 1 of every 9 deaths included HF as a diagnosis, reflecting 8% of the deaths attributable to cardiovascular disease (CVD).[1] It is estimated that by 2030, the total direct medical costs of HF will increase nearly 120%,[2] with associated CVD direct medical costs projected to reach more than $918 billion.[1] Although hospitalization is common for the patient population with HF, more than half of all admissions are for non-CVD-related causes.[3] The complexity of care for patients at the time of transition from the hospital to other settings requires resources, coordination, and the expertise of multiple members of the health care team.

CHANGES IN HEALTH CARE

Since the passage of the Affordable Care Act in 2010, a shift has occurred in health care professionals' thinking, and changes in the delivery models have emerged. These changes include a movement from private practice models to integrated delivery systems, a movement from an emphasis on acute care, procedure-driven reimbursement, to value-based bundling and fee structures based on capitation models, and delivery of population health, disease prevention, and chronic disease management models.[4]

The challenge facing health care professionals is how to best deliver the highest quality of care in the most efficient way, in particular in transitions of care. What does effective team-based care look like? Team-based HF care relies on members from many disciplines, including nurses, physicians, social workers, pharmacists, therapists, and behavioral health specialists. The 3 million nurses who coordinate care have been identified as key to high-quality evidence-based team care.[5]

The health care system is more sophisticated than ever before. Patients, as increasingly educated consumers of health care, are learning about, expecting, and experiencing this new delivery model all across the nation. As detailed in the *Wall Street Journal* just this year, an increasing number of physician practices are abandoning "the traditional 1-on-1 doctor-patient relationship."[6] As fee-for-service financial models are being abandoned and bundled payment structures are increasingly deployed,[7] team members are needed to contribute to the full extent and scope of their training and licensure.[5]

[a] Department of Surgery, Columbia University Medical Center, 21 Audubon Avenue, 2nd Floor, Room 209, New York, NY 14845, USA; [b] Frances Payne Bolton School of Nursing, Case Western Reserve University, 10900 Euclid Avenue, Cleveland, OH 44106, USA; [c] Department of Heart Failure and Cardiac Transplantation, St Vincent Heart Center of Indiana, 8333 Naab Road, Suite #400, Indianapolis, IN 46260, USA
* Corresponding author.
E-mail address: macwalsh@iquest.net

Heart Failure Clin 11 (2015) 371–378
http://dx.doi.org/10.1016/j.hfc.2015.03.003

EFFECTIVE HEALTH CARE TEAMS FOR CHRONIC CARE

Particularly in the vulnerable aging population, a team-based approach is most effective.[8] Complex information and interpersonal connections make it difficult for a single provider to render care in isolation and have the potential to be harmful. Clinicians working together can become a team, with the common goal of providing the best possible care.[9]

Although team-based care has shown tremendous value and many disease-specific examples have been effective,[10] the emergence of the core principles in highly performing transitional teams is still yet to be formalized or clearly defined. Although HF chronic disease teams,[11] cardiac transplantation,[12] operating room teams,[13] rapid response teams,[14] and hospice care[15] have been evaluated, lack of homogeneity and common terminology has hindered further interprofessional team research. Theoretic models are emerging that provide a potential framework applicable across various clinical settings, regions, and disciplines.[16]

However, the heterogeneity of team structures does not eliminate the need for establishment of core elements that support effective collaboration. Primarily, the focus must remain on patients and their needs as defined and determined by their personal priorities. In addition, essential clinical roles must be accounted for in every setting. Even although the formal title of the contributing members may change and the role of team leader may shift from setting to setting, the essentials must be met for the team to be effective. Again, the clinical members of the team must reflect variability, region by region, depending on the patient and clinical population.

GUIDING FRAMEWORK FOR TEAM-BASED CARE IN HEART FAILURE TRANSITIONS

Transitions of care for patients with HF are complex, because teams from the hospital, home care, skilled facility, and outpatient clinics are challenged to provide team-to-team communication and coordination without compensation. Team-based care provides health services to individuals, families, or their communities, using multiple health care providers, who work together with patients and their caregivers to accomplish shared goals, spanning health care settings to achieve coordinated high-quality care.[17] Aspects that support the effectiveness of team-based care include a shared focus (the patient), shared values, and shared principles.

Five personal values that were identified by Mitchell and colleagues[9] in the *Core Principles & Values of Effective Team-Based Health Care* as shared by high-functioning team members include honesty, discipline, creativity, humility, and curiosity.

Teams are the sum of their individual members and are unique in size, makeup, settings, and styles of communication. However, to be effective, they must adhere to established principles, which are identified shared goals, clear roles with well-defined expectations, earned mutual trust and mutual respect, effective communication that is prioritized and iterative in nature, as well as mutually agreed measurable processes and outcomes, with a process of feedback and performance improvement.[9] The team-based approach is not prescriptive but is founded on core values, principles, and standards that support effective collaboration.

Establishment of an organizing framework in development of effective team-based care is paramount. The group assembled at the Transitions of Care Consensus Conference (TOCCC)[18] accomplished much work, and lessons can be learned from the principles put forth by the Stepping Up to the Plate (SUTTP) Alliance of the American Board of Internal Medicine.[18] They established 5 principles of effective transitional care as accountability, communication, timely feedback and feedforward of information, involvement of the patient and family member, unless inappropriate in all steps, and respect of the hub of coordination of care.

The TOCCC added additional principles to those identified by the SUTTP and believed that opportunities remained. They added the following principles:

- Patients should have and be able to identify their medical home or coordinating practitioner.
- At each point of care, the patient and caregiver need to know who is primarily responsible for their care, whom to contact, and how to reach them.
- Transitional care national standards should be adopted and implemented at the national and community level.
- Standardized metrics for monitoring and improving transitions should be used for continuous quality improvement and accountability.[18]

The proposed standards for effective care transitions include coordinating clinicians, care plans, communication infrastructure, standard communication formats, transition responsibility, timeliness, community standards, and measurement.[18]

WHY TEAM-BASED TRANSITIONS OF CARE?

Research has taught us that we are better together.[19] When teams come together to focus on delivering the highest quality of care by enhancing each team member's contribution to the health care delivery process, the result is transformational for patients with HF. The goal is to focus care solely on the goals of the patient. Conceptually, this requires a high level of communication not only between clinicians but also between teams at different facilities during the transitions of care. The greatest benefit that a team brings to the patient is various assessment perspectives, listening styles, and specialized training.[20] However, when the team works cohesively and keeps the focus and goals of therapy on the patient, the approach should include the highest level of shared decision making, which supports the outcomes most relevant to each individual patient.

A highly functioning team approach goes beyond providing clinical options to patients and actively engages in productive discussions to produce the highest-quality outcomes in the context of the patient's values, goals, and overall preferences. In the current fee-for-service health care delivery model, patient education is often pushed to the nice-to-have column of care versus the essential components list. At transitions, patients and family members experience significant anxiety,[18] and the essential nature of dedicated, team-based, effective education is core to the ability to improve the quality of care.

HOSPITAL READMISSION

Approximately 20% of Medicare beneficiaries hospitalized for HF are readmitted within 30 days of hospital discharge. Because of the economic burden on the US health care system, the Patient Protection Affordable Care Act of 2010 created incentives to reduce readmissions. Section 3025 of the Affordable Care Act added section 1886(q) to the Social Security Act, establishing the Hospital Readmissions Reduction Program, which requires Centers for Medicare and Medicaid Services (CMS) to reduce payments to inpatient prospective payment system hospitals with excess readmissions.

An initial focus of CMS has been on those patients readmitted to hospitals with a discharge diagnosis of HF, myocardial infarction, and pneumonia. Hospitals are at risk of losing up to 3% of their Medicare reimbursement in 2015, and it is anticipated that reimbursement penalties will continue in the future, with broadening to include other diagnoses. In response to these penalties, hospitals have made readmission reduction a priority and readmission reduction has been the focus of national, state-based, and local quality campaigns and collaborations.

Prevention of Readmission

Evidence about how best to reduce HF readmissions is growing. Several randomized trials have reported discharge and follow-up interventions that reduced readmissions.[21–27] Efforts aimed at patient education,[28,29] early follow-up after discharge,[30] and comprehensive multidisciplinary discharge care[31] have each shown promise with regard to reduction of readmission (**Box 1**).

It is this promise, shown by efforts at multidisciplinary care, that has pushed forward interest in team-based transitions in care for patients with HF.[32] Additional benefits to comprehensive patient and family education include an enhanced patient experience related to effective communication and education, ensuring accurate medication reconciliation, verification of confirmed follow-up appointments, and improved hand-off communication to other providers.

Transitional Care Models

Health care transitions occur frequently. Patients transition between care settings, as well as between acute and chronic health care teams and practitioners. Transitional care must be a priority to improve outcomes and quality of care. The transitional care model, care transitions intervention, better outcomes for older adults through safe transitions, reengineered discharge, and interventions to reduce acute care transfers are examples of programs found to be effective to reduce avoidable hospital readmission and are described in the following sections.

TRANSITIONAL CARE MODEL

A multidisciplinary team of researchers from the University of Pennsylvania designed the transitional care model in 1980.[33] Originally developed for the transitional care of high-risk mothers and babies, the model was modified to address the specific needs of the elderly, chronically ill population. Core components of the transitional care model (TCM) include primary care coordinator or transitional care nurse, an in-hospital assessment, 24/7 support, regular follow-up, and education of patient, family, and informal caregivers.[34]

Box 1
Strategies to reduce readmission after hospital discharge

- Patient education
- Early follow-up
- Multidisciplinary disease management

With the goal of ensuring continuity of care across settings and clinicians, and improving outcomes in the at-risk patient, TCM is an evidence-based, advanced practice nurse-led, team-based model of care, which showed effectiveness. Patients' improvements included improved short-term quality of life, improved satisfaction with care, and fewer readmissions to hospital. In 3 National Institute of Nursing trials, the mean saving per patient was $5000.[33] The cost-effectiveness of intentional transitional care programs has been shown.[25] When intentional advanced practice nurse-delivered interventions in the elderly population with HF was examined, financial reward was shown (**Fig. 1**) as well as improved quality of life and patient satisfaction.[35]

CARE TRANSITIONS INTERVENTION

The care transitions program is a 4-week hospital to home program that uses a transitions coach, a role filled by trained lay community workers.[21] The primary areas of emphasis include medication self-management, a patient-generated, patient-centered record, encouragement of patient-managed/coordinated follow-up care, and patient understanding of symptoms and progression of disease. A randomized control trial reported that the patients who received the intervention had a lower rehospitalization rate at 30 and 90 days, as well as lower mean hospital costs at 180 days.[21]

BETTER OUTCOMES FOR OLDER ADULTS THROUGH SAFE TRANSITIONS

Developed as a quality improvement initiative by the Society of Hospital Medicine, the 5-key elements of this model include a comprehensive intervention, a comprehensive implementation

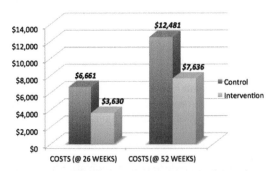

Fig. 1. Transitional care decreases costs. (*Data from* Naylor MD, Brooten D, Campbell R, et al. Comprehensive discharge planning and home follow-up of hospitalized elders. JAMA 1999;281:613–20; and Naylor MD, Brooten DA, Campbell RL, et al. Transitional care of older adults with heart failure: a randomized controlled trial. J Am Geriatr Soc 2004;52:675–84.)

guide, including detailed instructions and resources, ongoing program support, a collaborative network, and online resources. This program showed reduction in readmissions in participating institutions. Additional benefits included enhanced communications and perceived improvements in level of service by patients.[36]

REENGINEERED DISCHARGE

A group from Boston University Medical Center developed reengineered discharge (project RED).[37] A quality improvement project, RED incorporated 12 components, with a focus on discharge planning. Led by a specially trained discharge advocate, the core aspects include enhanced discharge planning, coordination and education, communication and transmission of discharge summary with outpatient providers, and early postdischarge follow-up calls for reinforcement of education and problem solving. The results included a significant reduction in hospital utilization by patients in the intervention group, showing the most effectiveness in those patients with the highest hospital utilization in the preceding 6 months.

INTERVENTIONS TO REDUCE ACUTE CARE TRANSFERS

Interventions to reduce acute care transfers (INTERACT) is a transitional care model that was developed to focus on the transition from nursing home to hospital.[38] A quality improvement program, INTERACT provides resources to skilled nursing facilities to reduce avoidable transfers to the acute care setting. Early recognition of changes in resident status, assessment, documentation, and timely interprofessional communication are key aspects of this model. Effective implementation by medical directors and primary care clinicians in the nursing home settings has been associated with a reduction in hospitalization of long-term residents.[38]

EVIDENCE FOR TRANSITIONAL CARE

Transitions are highly vulnerable episodes, which show clear safety and quality opportunities.[18] One study[39] found that 1 in 5 patients experienced an adverse event after discharge from an acute care facility. Adverse events were defined as medical management–associated injury, and this same study[18] reported that 66% of these events were drug related.

Transitional care interventions, for chronically ill patients being discharged from hospital to home, have shown their effectiveness[40] and have been associated with reduced readmission in the short-term, intermediate-term, and long-term. Care coordination by a nurse, implementing high-intensity interventions, was identified as most effective in reducing short-term readmission.[41]

Many randomized control trials have shown the effectiveness of transitional care programs, but not all. Two Canadian older adult programs failed to show success. A low intervention dose such as a single home visit followed by telephone follow-up is a potential rationale for unsuccessful programs.[42,43] The high-risk, chronically ill population was the focus of most studies reviewed by Naylor and colleagues.[33] Vulnerable groups, those who are a focus of the Affordable Care Acts provisions, are particularly absent from the research, showing a knowledge gap and opportunity for future study.[41]

THE NAVIGATOR MODEL: ENHANCING TEAM-BASED TRANSITIONS

The patient navigator model initially emerged in 1990 in response to the needs of patients with cancer. Developed to address common barriers experienced by newly diagnosed patients to support access and timeliness of care, this model subsequently evolved to apply across the continuum of care.[44] Program momentum continued when the National Cancer Institute established funding for the implementation and evaluation of patient navigator programs in cancer care in 2002.[45] The promising results from these early navigation examples lend themselves to the spread of the concept to other complex and chronic disease management programs. With the overarching theme of removing barriers and improving patient outcomes and quality of care, patient navigation has been shown to be effective, with enhanced patient access to screenings and improving survival rates.[46] The patient navigator model emphasizes continuity and coordination and ideally is a constant for the patient across the delivery system and continuum of care.

Transitions of care in the population with HF, as with other chronically ill patients, are a highly vulnerable period, which makes the role of the patient navigator pivotal. Navigating the ever-evolving health care delivery system is like traveling unknown highways, which without much warning can have new turns, potholes, and construction. With a patient navigator to partner the patient and family throughout the journey,[47] the potential benefits have a broad reach and the patient experience of care may be enhanced (**Fig. 2**).

Eliminating barriers, being a consistent presence and advocate, and enhancing

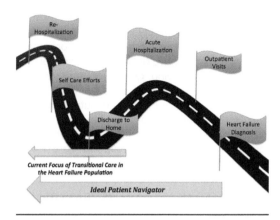

Fig. 2. Patient navigator.

communication across multiple teams and clinicians support not only establishment of an evidence-based plan of care for the patient but enhance the patient's ability to adhere to the plan.[46] Although historically most navigator programs have been initiated as a band-aid response to a difficult system that proves itself particularly challenging for the less fortunate, in the future, as financial compensation is increasingly supportive of team-based care and navigator programs, the concept of introducing a patient navigator at the time of HF diagnosis could be a game changer. If we could accelerate the initiation of the team development earlier in the patient experience of care, versus at the time of first acute care hospitalization or later, we could further improve outcomes, quality of life, and cost-effectiveness of care.

As shown in **Fig. 3**, the team-based approach and effectiveness of the team may be enhanced when patients with HF partner a navigator. Patient

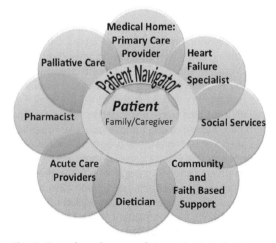

Fig. 3. Team-based approach to patient navigation.

navigation models, programs, and services continue to grow in many facets of health care.[47] As we build effective team-based HF programs, patient navigators have potential to show their significance in improving quality of care as they bridge the gap between HF teams at the hospital, home care, skilled nursing, and outpatient facilities. This role has great promise, and as navigator models continue to evolve, their role coordinating acute care teams with the chronic care teams should not be underestimated.

TEAM-BASED HEART FAILURE TRANSITION INITIATIVES

As part of its quality portfolio, the American College of Cardiology (ACC) has developed initiatives and tool kits to support clinicians in developing effective transitional care programs, specifically for the population with HF. The ACC has shown leadership in this arena by encouraging a multidisciplinary approach to treating HF, with the goal of improving the quality of care and health care efficiency and reducing unnecessary HF readmissions. Two programs that emphasize the implementation of a team-based approach to transitional care are hospital to home (H2H) and the patient navigator program (PNP).

H2H is a quality campaign sponsored by the ACC and Institute of Healthcare Improvement. Initially established with the goal of reducing readmission rates by 20% by the end of 2012, the program has secured more than 1500 hospital participants. The focus of the H2H program has been 3-fold and includes early follow-up after discharge, medication management, and patient signs. Most institutions participating in H2H reported having a quality improvement team in place to address HF readmissions specifically.[48]

The PNP is specifically designed to focus on the unique needs of patients discharged after hospitalization for HF or myocardial infarction. With the goal of developing a culture of patient centeredness during the vulnerable period after discharge, this program encourages the team approach to care by engaging with administrators, physicians, and nurses.[49]

Both programs were developed to support teams committed to improving transitional care. Hospitals that are participating in these programs test new approaches and enhance existing methods, sharing their learning. Since its inception in 2009, the H2H initiative has shown effectiveness, with 49% of participants reporting that their readmission rates had improved since their enrollment.[48] The PNP was implemented in 2014. The PNP will support 35 participating hospitals in the development of scalable team-based strategies and testing of new approaches to improve transitional care for populations with HF and myocardial infarction.

SUMMARY

With the implementation of the Patient Protection and Affordable Care Act, the requisite for health care systems to build team-based transitional care programs is clear. The clinical course for patients with HF is complicated and progressive, which leads to frequent acute care hospitalization and higher mortality. These patients uniquely benefit from transitions of care programs that encourage a coordinated, multidisciplinary team-based approach to care. Evidence of the benefit of this approach to care is mounting. Research and advocacy efforts need to continue to facilitate the team-based approach to transitions and improve the quality of care.

REFERENCES

1. Go AS, Mozaffarian D, Roger VL, et al. Heart disease and stroke statistics–2014 update a report from the American Heart Association. Circulation 2014;129(3):e28–292.
2. Go AS, Mozaffarian D, Roger VL, et al. Heart disease and stroke statistics 2013 update: a report from the American Heart Association. Circulation 2013;127(1):e6–245.
3. Deasi AS. Influence of hospitalization for cardiovascular versus noncardiovascular reasons on subsequent mortality in patients with chronic heart failure across the spectrum of ejection fraction. Circ Heart Fail 2014;7(6):895–902.
4. American Hospital Association. Workforce roles in a redesigned primary care model. 2013.
5. Institute of Medicine (US). Committee on the Robert Wood Johnson Foundation Initiative on the Future of Nursing. The future of nursing: leading change. Advancing health–Institute of Medicine. National Academies Press, 2011.
6. Landro L. The doctor's team will see you now. Wall St J 2014. Available at: http://online.wsj.com/articles/sb 10001424052702304899704579389203539061082.
7. Sanghavi D, George M, Bleibery S, et al. Treating congestive heart failure and the role of payment reform. Washington, DC: Brookings. The Merkin Series on Innovation in Care Delivery; 2014. p. 1–35.
8. Enderlin CA, McLeskey N, Rooker JL, et al. Review of current conceptual models and frameworks to guide transitions of care in older adults. Geriatr Nurs 2013;34(1):47–52.
9. Mitchell PH, Wynia MK, Golden R, et al. Core principles & values of effective team-based health care. Washington, DC: Institute of Medicine; 2012.

10. Naylor MD. Transitional care model. Nursing leadership. New York: Springer Publishing Company, 2011. Available at: ezproxy.cul.columbia.edu/login?qurl=http://literati.credoreference.com/content/entry/spnurld/transitional_care_model/0. Accessed November 24, 2014.

11. Savard LA, Thompson DR, Clark AM. A meta-review of evidence on heart failure disease management programs: the challenges of describing and synthesizing evidence on complex interventions. Trials 2011;12(1):194.

12. Jessup M, Albert NM, Lanfear DE, et al. ACCF/AHA/HFSA 2011 survey results: current staffing profile of heart failure programs, including programs that perform heart transplant and mechanical circulatory support device implantation: a report of the ACCF Heart Failure and Transplant Committee, AHA Heart Failure and Transplantation Committee, and Heart Failure Society of America. Circ Heart Fail 2011; 4(3):378–87.

13. Weaver SJ, Rosen MA, DizGranados D, et al. Does teamwork improve performance in the operating room? A multilevel evaluation. Jt Comm J Qual Patient Saf 2010;36:133–42.

14. Chan PS, Jain R, Nallmothu BK, et al. Rapid response teams: a systematic review and meta-analysis. JAMA 2010;170(1):18–26.

15. Hearn J, Higginson I. Do specialist palliative care teams improve outcomes for cancer patients? A systematic literature review. Palliat Med 1998;12(5): 317–32.

16. Core competencies for interprofessional collaborative practice: report of an expert panel. Washington, DC: Interprofessional Education Collaborative; 2011. Available at: http://www.aacn.nche.edu/education-resources/ipecreport.pdf.

17. Naylor MD, Coburn KD, Kutzman ET. Interprofessional team-based primary care for chronically ill adults: state of the science. Unpublished white paper presented at ABIM Foundation meeting to advance team-based care for the chronically ill in ambulatory settings. Philadelphia, PA, March 24–25, 2010.

18. Snow V, Beck D, Budnitz T, et al. Transitions of care consensus policy statement American College of Physicians–Society of General Internal Medicine-Society of Hospital Medicine–American Geriatrics Society–American College of Emergency Physicians–Society of Academic Emergency Medicine. J Hosp Med 2009;4(6):364–70.

19. Zwarenstein M, Goldman J, Reeves S. Interprofessional collaboration: effects of practice-based interventions on professional practice and healthcare outcomes. Cochrane Database Syst Rev 2009;(3):CD000072.

20. Lawson A, Hageman H, Rotter B, et al. Appreciation of interprofessional perspectives: a standardized patient experience to promote communication between nursing and medical students. 2013. Available at: https://www.mededportal.org/publication/9346. Accessed December 03, 2014.

21. Coleman EA. The care transitions intervention: results of a randomized controlled trial. Arch Intern Med 2006;166(17):1822–8.

22. Koehler BE, Richter KM, Youngblood L, et al. Reduction of 30-day postdischarge hospital readmission or emergency department (ED) visit rates in high-risk elderly medical patients through delivery of a targeted care bundle. J Hosp Med 2009;4(4): 211–8.

23. McDonald K, Ledwidge M, Cahill J, et al. Elimination of early rehospitalization in a randomized, controlled trial of multidisciplinary care in a high-risk, elderly heart failure population: the potential contributions of specialist care, clinical stability and optimal angiotensin-converting enzyme inhibitor dose at discharge. Eur J Heart Fail 2001;3(2):209–15.

24. Naylor M, Brooten D, Jones R, et al. Comprehensive discharge planning for the hospitalized elderly: a randomized clinical trial. Ann Intern Med 1994;120: 999–1006.

25. Naylor MD, Brooten D, Campbell R, et al. Comprehensive discharge planning and home follow-up of hospitalized elders: a randomized clinical trial. JAMA 1999;281(7):613–20.

26. Rainville EC. Impact of pharmacist interventions on hospital readmissions for heart failure. Am J Health Syst Pharm 1999;56(15):1339–42. Available at: http://www.ajhp.org/content/56/13/1339.citation.

27. Rich MW, Beckham V, Wittenberg C, et al. A multidisciplinary intervention to prevent the readmission of elderly patients with congestive heart failure. N Engl J Med 1995;333:1190–5. Available at: http://www.nejm.org/doi/full/10.1056/nejm199511023331806.

28. Krumholz HM, Amatruda J, Smith GL, et al. Randomized trial of an education and support intervention to prevent readmission of patients with heart failure. J Am Coll Cardiol 2002;39(1):83–9.

29. Koelling TM. Discharge education improves clinical outcomes in patients with chronic heart failure. Circulation 2005;111(2):179–85.

30. Hernandez AF, Greiner MA, Fonarow GC, et al. Relationship between early physician follow-up and 30-day readmission among Medicare beneficiaries hospitalized for heart failure. JAMA 2010;303(17): 1716–22.

31. Phillips CO, Wright SM, Kern DE, et al. Comprehensive discharge planning with postdischarge support for older patients with congestive heart failure: a metaanalysis. JAMA 2004;291:1358–67.

32. Schell W. A review: discharge navigation and its effect on heart failure readmissions. Prof Case Manag 2014;19:224–34.

33. Naylor MD, Aiken LH, Kurtzman ET, et al. The importance of transitional care in achieving health reform. Health Aff 2011;30(4):746–54.

34. Boutwell A, Griffin F, Hwu S, et al. Effective interventions to reduce rehospitalizations: a compendium of 15 promising interventions. Cambridge (MA): Institute for Healthcare Improvement; 2009.

35. Naylor MD, Brooten DA, Campbell RL, et al. Transitional care of older adults hospitalized with heart failure: a randomized, controlled trial. J Am Geriatr Soc 2004;52(5):675–84.

36. Project BOOST seeks to improve care transitions. Medical ethics advisor. AHC Media L.L.C. High-Beam Research. 2009. Available at: http://www.highbeam.com. Accessed December 10, 2014.

37. Malcolm G. Re-engineered discharge cuts readmissions. Hospital Case Management 2012;20(5):70–5.

38. Ouslander JG, Bonner A, Herndon L, et al. The interventions to reduce acute care transfers (INTERACT) quality improvement program: an overview for medical directors and primary care clinicians in long term care ouslander. J Am Med Dir Assoc 2014; 15(3):162–70.

39. Forster AJ. The incidence and severity of adverse events affecting patients after discharge from the hospital. Ann Intern Med 2003;138(3):161.

40. Stamp K, Machado M, Allen N. Transitional care programs improve outcomes for heart failure patients: an integrative review. J Cardiovasc Nurs 2014;29: 140–54.

41. Verhaegh K, MacNeil-Vroomen J, Eslami S, et al. Transitional care interventions prevent hospital readmissions for adults with chronic illnesses. Health Aff (Millwood) 2014;33(9):1531–9. Available at: http://content.healthaffairs.org/content/33/9/1531.full.html.

42. Gagnon AJ, Schein C, McVey L, et al. Randomized controlled trial of nurse case management of frail older people. J Am Geriatr Soc 1999;47(9):1118–24.

43. Dalby DM, Sellers JW, Fraser FD, et al. Effects of preventive home visits by a nurse on the outcomes of frail elderly people in the community: a randomized controlled trial. Can Med Assoc J 2000; 162(4):497–500.

44. Freeman HP, Rodriguez RL. History and principles of patient navigation. Cancer 2011;117:3537–40.

45. Robinson-White SR, Conroy B, Slavish K, et al. Patient navigation in breast cancer: a systematic review. Cancer Nurs 2010;33:127–40.

46. The most important healthcare job you've never heard of how patient navigation can improve health outcomes. 2012. Available at: http://www.himss.org/files/himssorg/content/files/accenture_pov_accenture_most_important.pdf. Accessed December 03, 2014.

47. Palos G, Hare M. Patients, family caregivers, and patient navigators: a partnership approach. Cancer 2011;117:3592–602.

48. Bradley EH, Curry L, Horwitz LI, et al. Hospital strategies associated with 30-day readmission rates for patients with heart failure. Circ Cardiovasc Qual Outcomes 2013;6(4):444–50.

49. ACC Patient Navigator Program. CardioSource. Available at: http://cvquality.acc.org/Initiatives/Patient-Navigator.aspx. Acessed December 03, 2014.

Team-Based Care for Outpatients with Heart Failure

Julie W. Creaser, MN*, Eugene C. DePasquale, MD,
Elizabeth Vandenbogaart, MSN, Darlene Rourke, MSN,
Tamara Chaker, MSN, Gregg C. Fonarow, MD

KEYWORDS

- Disease management • Multidisciplinary heart failure team
- Outpatient heart failure medical therapy • Telemonitoring • Advanced care options

KEY POINTS

- Concentrated, team-based outpatient heart failure programs may be able to provide more focused care that could improve the quality of care and patient-center outcomes.
- There has been a growing recognition of the role of team-based care for enhancing the management of heart failure.
- Implementing team-based care for outpatients with heart failure significantly reduces rehospitalization and cost, and improves functional status and quality of life.
- Effective and safe use and optimization of guideline-directed therapy are critical in reducing mortality and rehospitalization.

INTRODUCTION

Heart failure (HF) is a concerning health care problem associated with significant morbidity, mortality, and costs. There are approximately 825,000 new HF cases annually. An estimated 5.1 million Americans older than 20 years have HF. Eighty percent of patients with HF are elderly (≥65 years). In 2010, there were 676,000 emergency department (ED) visits and 236,000 outpatient visits with an estimated 1,801,000 physician office visits having the primary diagnosis of HF. Projections show that the prevalence of HF will increase 46% from 2012 to 2030, resulting in more than 8 million Americans older than 18 years with HF. Survival with HF has improved over time, but mortality remains high at 50% at 5 years.[1–3]

Furthermore, the diagnosis of HF carries a tremendous financial burden, with an estimated cost of $30.7 billion annually. The annual cost of HF will increase considerably to an estimated $69.7 billion by 2030.[3–5] HF treatment costs can be divided into several major components. In the United States in-hospital care is responsible for 60% of HF-related costs[6] while regular outpatient follow-up by general physicians, cardiologists, and/or specialized HF nurses and chronic medication are far lower.

The rising costs are in part due to patients with HF living longer because of the increased use of guideline-directed medical therapy (GDMT), development of advanced strategies for outpatient HF disease management, and other life-prolonging

Dr G.C. Fonarow reports consulting with Amgen, Bayer, Gambro, Janssen, Novartis, and Medtronic. The other authors have no disclosures or conflicts of interest.
Division of Cardiology, Department of Medicine, Ahmanson-UCLA Cardiomyopathy Center, University of California, 100 UCLA Medical Plaza, Suite 630 East, Los Angeles, CA 90095, USA
* Corresponding author. Ahmanson-UCLA Cardiomyopathy Center, Ronald Reagan UCLA Medical Center, 100 Medical Plaza, Suite 630 East, Los Angeles, CA 90095.
E-mail address: jcreaser@mednet.ucla.edu

Heart Failure Clin 11 (2015) 379–405
http://dx.doi.org/10.1016/j.hfc.2015.03.004
1551-7136/15/$ – see front matter © 2015 Elsevier Inc. All rights reserved.

therapies such as devices (ie, implantable-cardioverter defibrillator [ICD], mechanical circulatory support [MCS]) with proven impact on morbidity and mortality.[6,7] Owing to the prevalence and rising costs, a variety of outpatient team–based HF management programs have been created over the past few decades. With the high volume of patients, HF clinics in the ambulatory care setting are in demand and their numbers continue to grow. These clinics treat the spectrum of HF from acute episodes to chronic management in outpatient settings. Clinics were designed to improve HF-related outcomes by decreasing readmissions and increasing survival.[8,9] Programs that apply team-based multidisciplinary care were consistently superior to that supplied by just an individual.[10,11]

Team-Based Care for Outpatients with Heart Failure

Improving outpatient HF management comes with significant responsibility to patients and health care systems. Practitioners who treat patients with HF are challenged to manage numerous comorbidities requiring multiple medications and lifestyle changes in an older, sometimes cognitively and psychologically affected patient group. Hospital readmissions or worsening HF symptoms are often preventable, and have been associated with modifiable factors such as insufficient use of GDMT, poor medication adherence, and poor adherence to fluid or salt restriction.[12–14] As a result, several initiatives were started to address and overcome the challenges in outpatient HF management.[15] Team care has generally been embraced by most as a criterion for high-quality care.[16] A multidisciplinary team-based approach to health care has been recognized for more than a decade as providing value through comprehensive, integrative management that encompasses use of best practices, clinical practice improvement, information technology, patient-centered outcomes, and chronic disease management. The goal of the interdisciplinary team is to deliver safe, effective, cost-containing, and culturally and linguistically appropriate interventions within and across care settings.[17–19]

Disease management programs (DMPs) were born out of the necessity for a multidisciplinary framework for treatment of chronic diseases that required complex medical and socioeconomic considerations.[20] Essential attributes, as suggested by the American Heart Association (AHA) Disease Management Taxonomy Writing Group, included clearly defined use of individualized, disease-targeted, evidence-based guideline interventions delivered through multidisciplinary

team care, comprehensive patient education, medication management with consideration for environment, method, delivery, intensity, and frequency of communication with providers, and assessment of outcomes measures (**Table 1**).[20,21] Furthermore, national HF guideline writers recommended a team model of care to facilitate adherence to evidence-based practices and outlined key components of an HF DMP.[22,23] HF DMPs typically include 3 overlapping components: HF clinics, home care, and telemonitoring, or a combination of these methods (**Fig. 1**).[15,18,24]

The specialized HF clinic has become a vital element in comprehensive care and chronic management in outpatient settings for patients by practitioners with expertise in HF. Patients' management plans are formulated through an integrated multidisciplinary team approach beginning with patients and caregivers/family members.[18]

The earliest description of specialized HF clinics was in 1983.[25] However, greater development did not take significant shape until a landmark pilot study by Rich and colleagues[26,27] in 1993 when they demonstrated fewer hospital readmissions and a decreased number of hospital days in the HF multidisciplinary intervention group.[28] Later studies implementing team-based HF clinic interventions also reported improved functional status, quality of life, and HF medication optimization, and reduction in hospital readmissions, length of hospital stay, and health care costs.[29–37] Reduction in mortality and HF hospitalizations were further supported by subsequent meta-analyses evaluating HF clinic care in comparison with usual care.[28,38–40]

A systematic review of 29 randomized trials (5039 patients) incorporating multidisciplinary strategies for HF management reported reduced mortality, HF hospitalizations, and all-cause hospitalizations.[41] Furthermore, improving patient self-care reduced hospitalizations but not mortality, although strategies that used telephone contact with referral to primary care physicians reduced only HF hospitalizations. Multidisciplinary strategies saved costs in 15 of 18 trials that evaluated cost-effectiveness.[20,41] A meta-analysis by Whelan and colleagues[40] demonstrated that hospitalizations (HF and all-cause) and length of stay in hospital were decreased if patients attended follow-up with a cardiologist; this was not demonstrated with general internist management (see **Table 1**; **Table 2**).[42]

Home-Based Programs

In a home-based model, care is provided through home visits, telephone monitoring, or both. Home

Table 1
Selective studies of outpatient heart failure clinics

Reference	Sample	Study Design	Intervention	Components of Intervention	Outcomes
Multidisciplinary HF Clinic Interventions					
Cintron et al,[25] 1983	15 NYHA III–IV, mean age 65 y Sex of patients not indicated although study conducted at a Veteran's Administration hospital so likely exclusively men Puerto Rico	Within-subjects preintervention, postintervention comparison with mean follow-up of 24 mo	HF clinic staffed with nurse practitioners	Nurse practitioner managed Frequent follow-up via clinic visits Education reinforced at each visit: medication, weight control, diet Assessment of home situation Family support Increased availability of nurse practitioner ("walk-ins" encouraged) Cardiologist consultation for unstable patients	60% reduction in rehospitalizations 85% reduction in hospital days Reduction in total medical costs of $8009.00 per patient
Lasater,[29] 1996	41 HF patients USA	Within-subjects preintervention, postintervention comparison with mean follow-up of 6 and 12 mo	HF clinic staffed by APNs	Four weekly visits with an experienced hospital staff nurse Direct access to physician consultation, social worker, dietician Patient education regarding diuretic regimen and importance of daily weights Scales provided as needed Diuretics adjusted based on physical assessment Medication compliance monitored Assistance with financial constraints	4% decrease in readmission rate Mean hospital length of stay decreased 1.6 d Increased knowledge of medical regimen demonstrated at 1 y

(continued on next page)

Table 1
(continued)

Reference	Sample	Study Design	Intervention	Components of Intervention	Outcomes
Hanumanthu et al,[60] 1997	134 NYHA not indicated, mean age 52 ± 12 y 71% male USA	Within-subjects preintervention, postintervention comparison with follow-up of 12 mo	Physician-directed, nurse-coordinated comprehensive HF clinic	HF/transplant physician directed Nurse coordinators assisted with inpatient and outpatient management Team exclusively managed HF patients Optimization of medical therapy Periodic meetings with home health care agency and hospice program to integrate care	53% reduction in annual hospitalization rate 63% reduction in HF rehospitalizations Increased peak Vo_2
Fonarow et al,[61] 1997	214 NYHA III and IV, mean age 52 ± 10 y 81% male USA	Within-subjects preintervention, postintervention comparison with follow-up of 6 mo	HF cardiologist directed, APN, follow-up, comprehensive inpatient and outpatient management program	HF cardiologist directed Follow-up by HF cardiologist, APN, and referring physician Optimization of drug therapy in hospital and during follow-up Comprehensive patient and family/caregiver education by HF clinical nurse specialist about daily weights and flexible diuretic regimen, diet, medications, smoking and alcohol abstinence, home exercise instruction, warning signs of worsening HF, and prognosis Weekly follow-up at HF clinic until stable with education reinforced Phone follow-up after medication changes and if indicated	85% reduction in rehospitalizations Improvement in functional status Lower costs

Study	N	Patient characteristics	Study design	Intervention	Description	Outcomes
Smith et al,[30] 1997	21	Mean NYHA 2.6 ± 0.5, mean age 61 y, 100% male, USA	Within-subjects preintervention, postintervention comparison with follow-up of 6 mo	Physician or nurse practitioner comprehensive care in HF clinic	Care provided by physician or nurse practitioner; Optimization of medical therapy; Identification and management of etiology of HF; Patient education about diet, medications, compliance, daily weights and flexible diuretic regimen, alcohol abstinence; Nurse practitioner available by phone; Increased access to clinic (without appointment) for worsening symptoms or medication needs	86% reduction in HF hospitalizations; Improved QOL; Improved functional status; More patients on optimal medications and doses
Cline et al,[31] 1998	190	Mean NYHA 2.6 ± 0.7, mean age 75.6 ± 5.3 y, 52.3% male, Sweden	RCT with follow-up of 12 mo	Nurse-directed outpatient clinic	Before hospital discharge, patient and family education about HF and pharmacologic and nonpharmacologic aspects of its treatment; Medication organizer given; Patients receive guidelines for self-management of diuretics; One-hour information visits for patient and family at home after discharge; Easy access to a nurse-directed outpatient clinic with one prescheduled visit at 8 mo; nurses available by phone and could see patients at short notice; Encouragement to contact nurses at clinic for any problems or questions or concerns	Time to first admission 33% longer in intervention group; 59% increase in no. of days hospitalized compared with 12 mo period before start of study in control group vs no increase in intervention group; 36% fewer hospitalizations in intervention group (but nonsignificant at $P = .08$); Trend toward mean annual reduction in health care costs ($P = .07$) per pt $1300 for IG (CG $3594 vs $2294 IG)

(continued on next page)

Table 1
(continued)

Reference	Sample	Study Design	Intervention	Components of Intervention	Outcomes
Dahl & Penque,[32] 2000	1192 nonrandomized patients (583 before program, 609 after program initiated) Pretreatment group mean age 72 y, 95% Caucasian Posttreatment group mean age 75 y, 96% Caucasian USA	Posttest only design with nonequivalent groups	APN-directed inpatient HF program	APN-coordinated inpatient care Intensive patient education HF medical orders reviewed with primary physician in reference to clinical guidelines Multidisciplinary services as needed Home health care plan High risk patients telephoned after discharge	36% reduction in hospital deaths Increased ACE inhibitor use Decreased 90 d HF readmission rates (14.6% to 8.4%) Shorter length of hospital stay (6.1 to 5.3 d/patient)
McDonald et al,[33] 2002	98 Age 70.80 ± 10.47 y Male 66.3% NYHA 2.29 ± 0.63 LVEF (%) 38.1 ± 12.6 High-risk HF patients Ireland	RCT; study duration 3 mo	Inpatient to outpatient HF clinic Physician, HF nurses, dietician optimization of therapy and achievement of clinical stability in both groups For IG: education of patient and family by HF nurse, dietary consultation (dietician), multiple visits during index admission	Weekly telephone calls by the HF nurse for 12 wk: evaluation of clinical status and education Enhancement, self-care HF clinic visits twice by patients and next of kin: clinical review, optimization of pharmacotherapy, weight control, intravenous diuretic when needed	Significant differences in HF readmission rates (25.5% IG vs 3.9% CG; P<.01) Readmission RR 0.31 At 3 mo death/readmission for HF 25.5% routine care vs 7.8% IG/multidisciplinary care Superior knowledge of HF medications and diet in IG, sustained at 3 mo

Study	Patients	Design	Setting	Intervention	Outcomes
Atienza et al,[34] 2004	338 Median age 68 (IQR: 59–74) y Male 60% NYHA I–IV LVEF (%): CG:42 ± 13, IG: 40 ± 15 Spain	RCT; study duration 12 mo	Inpatient to outpatient HF clinic Physician, HF nurse coordinated Education of patient and family by cardiac nurse: self-care enhancement, advice for diuretic self-adjustment, symptom management, teaching brochure Interview to detect possible factors that could lead to poor outcomes	Single home visit by physician 2 wk postdischarge, follow-up visits in HF clinic every 3 mo to enhance treatment adherence and knowledge, optimization of therapy. Nurse-coordinated visits to other specialists. Telephone contact available through telephone communication monitor (24-hourly) or by calling the HF clinic	All-cause readmission rates reduced in IG vs CG by 37% per 100 patients, (P<.001) and HF readmission rates reduced by 30% per 100 patients (P<.001) QOL improved Overall cost of care reduction in IG
Thompson et al,[35] 2005	106 Mean age 72 y 72% male LVEF (%) ≤45 UK	RCT; study duration 6 mo	Inpatient to outpatient HF clinic Nurse-led HF clinic HF nurse visit before discharge: discharge planning	Single home visit: education of patient and family and clinical examination Nurse available on phone during working hours Monthly visits to nurse-led HF clinic for at least 6 mo: full education package, clinical examination, treatment overview, and spironolactone introduction according to guidelines	Significantly fewer unplanned readmissions in IG (15 vs 45: P<.01)
Del Sindaco et al,[36] 2007	173 Mean age 70 y Male 52% NYHA II–IV Italy	RCT; study duration 24 mo	Physician-directed Hospital HF clinics (cardiologist and HF nurse) and home based (GP visits) Education and discharge planning	Education and educational booklet, weight charts, optimization of therapy, improved communication with health care providers, symptom management, adherence assessment, hospital clinic visits for continued education and therapy optimization (cardiologist), telephone follow-up, home visits by general practitioner with decreased frequency	Reduced number of HF readmission (−39.7%, P = .003) and all-cause readmission (−29.1%, P = .014) compared with CG Reduced no. of hospital days Pt reported significant improvement in functional status, QOL Cost-effective mean saving $982.04 per pt

(continued on next page)

Table 1
(continued)

Reference	Sample	Study Design	Intervention	Components of Intervention	Outcomes
Jaarsma et al,[37] 2008	1023 Mean age 71 y Male 62% NYHA I–IV LVEF (%) 34 ± 14 (SD) Netherlands	RCT; study duration 18 mo duration	Multicenter 3 groups CG cardiologist IG #1 basic support group and IG #2 intensive support group: education and support by HF nurse, self-care enhancement	Basic support group: HF clinic visits, further education, nurse telephonically available Intensive support group: all the above plus monthly contact with the nurse, weekly telephone calls, 2 home visits, multidisciplinary advice (dietician, social worker, physiotherapist)	No statistically significant differences in readmissions (HF and all-cause) between groups Not statistically significant: 15% reduction in mortality in IG

Multidisciplinary Home/Telephone Interventions

Reference	Sample	Study Design	Intervention	Components of Intervention	Outcomes
Rich et al,[26] 1995	282 Mean age 79 y Male 37% NYHA CG: 2. 4± 1.1, IG: 2.4 ± 1.0 High-risk HF patients USA	RCT; study duration 3 mo	Inpatient to outpatient Home telephone follow-up Education of patient and family, booklet, multidisciplinary interventions (dietician, social service consultation), discharge planning by cardiac nurse, medication adjustment by geriatric cardiologists	Telephone follow-up and home visits to review medications, enhance education and compliance with medication and diet, deterioration detection	Number of HF readmissions was reduced by 56.2% in IG ($P = .04$). No significant reductions for all-cause readmissions Because of decrease in hospital admissions, overall cost of care $460 less/pt in IG Subgroup of 126 pts: QOL scores at 90 d improved from baseline in IG ($P = .001$)
Stewart et al,[51] 1999	200 Mean age 76 y Male 48% NYHA II–IV at discharge Australia	RCT; study duration 6 mo	Nurse-led home visits Follow-up with cardiologist, PCP	Nurse-led education, counseling, exercise regimen Home visit 7–14 d after discharge Assessment regarding need for medication adjustment per protocol Telephone contact at 3 and 6 mo	All-cause readmissions 42% lower in IG Fewer associated days in hospital in IG (460 vs 1173; $P = .02$) Reduced costs

Study	Patients	Design	Intervention team	Intervention	Outcomes
Blue et al,[47] 2001	165 Mean age CG: 75.6 (SD 7.9), IG: 74.4 (SD 8.6) y Male CG 41%, IG: 54% NYHA II–IV UK	RCT; study duration 12 mo	Home visits Nurse-led, physician, pharmacist, social worker	First visit in hospital then 2 wk after discharge Home visits of decreased frequency for: education, self-care empowerment, booklet, medication and therapy optimization, liaison with other professions, telephone follow-up (nurse specialist) as needed Psychological support, protocol-driven medication titration	Fewer all-cause (86 vs 114, $P = .018$) and HF readmissions (19 vs 45, $P<.001$) in IG compared with CG. Risk of HF readmission reduced by 62% in IG Fewer days in hospital for HF in IG (mean 3.43 vs 7.46 d; $P = .0051$)
Riegel et al,[53] 2002	358 Mean age 74 y Male 59% NYHA >III 97% USA	RCT; study duration 6 mo	Nurse case management Nurse telephone support, liaison with PCP	Nurse telephone contact (median 14 calls), patient education and counseling, case management guided by computer decision support	Readmission (all-cause or HF) RR 0.53, $P = .01$ HF hospitalization rate was 45% lower ($P = .03$) in IG at 3 mo and 47.8% lower ($P = .01$) at 6 mo Higher degree of patient satisfaction
Laramee et al,[54] 2003	287 Mean age 70.7 y Male CG: 50%, IG: 58% NYHA I–IV LVEF (%) <40 USA	RCT; study duration 3 mo	Telephone support Nurse case manager provided discharge planning, education, self-care enhancement coordination of care between other professions: social workers, physical therapists, and dieticians	Booklet, self-care diary, weight and medication lists given before discharge Nurse-initiated telephone calls (10) for 12 wk long, further education of patient and promotion of optimal pharmacotherapy, nurse available on phone until home visit Case manager sent reminders to primary care physician if not on target medications	No significant difference in all-cause and HF readmissions Significantly lower readmissions in IG vs CG in a subgroup of pts ($P = .03$): pts who lived locally and saw a cardiologist Total inpt and outpt median costs and readmission median costs were reduced, 14% and 26% for IG

(continued on next page)

Table 1
(continued)

Reference	Sample	Study Design	Intervention	Components of Intervention	Outcomes
Naylor et al,[55] 2004	239 Mean age 76 y Male 43% LVEF: 25%–34%: 56% CG, 57% IG USA	RCT; 3 mo intervention, 13 mo follow-up	Home visits Visits nurse specialist (APN) before patient's discharge: education, discharge planning, transition actions	Nurse Specialist (APN): at least 8 home visits for educating patient and family, clinical evaluation, medication adjustment, visits during readmissions, telephone availability, collaboration with other professions, motivation for applying self-care practices	Significantly fewer total readmissions in IG (P = .047; 1 y) Lower mean total costs ($7636 vs $12,481, P = .002) Short-term improvement: QOL (12 wk P<.05)
Anderson et al,[56] 2005	121 Mean age 78.5 y Male 38% NYHA I–III USA	RCT; study duration 6 mo	Home visits Cardiac nurse: individualized education and discharge planning, written information, diet and activity plan by dietician and physiotherapist, scale provided	6-wk home care by cardiac trained community nurses (6–20 visits) to empower self-care, telephone follow-up for patient evaluation after 2 wk (nurse case manager), liaison with physician when needed	HF readmission rates were reduced near to 75% in IG compared with CG (P<.01) Average total cost saving for each subject in IG was $1541. Cost to implement program $158/pt
Kwok et al,[162] 2008	105 Mean age CG: 76.8 ± 7.0; IG: 79.5 ± 6.6 y Male 45% LVEF <40% CG: 30%, IG: 18% (for 12 patients not reported) China	RCT; study duration 6 mo	Home visits Community nurse visit at hospital before discharge: counseling, education, self-care enhancement	Home visits by CN in descending frequency: clinical evaluation, compliance enhancement evaluation, advice, social support if needed or either telephone call to monitor subjects who refused home visits, nurse available through bagger, nurse visit in case of readmission, liaison with doctors	No significant differences in readmission rates (P = .233), median no. of readmission tended to be lower in IG

Abbreviations: ACE, angiotensin-converting enzyme; APN, advanced practice nurse; CG, control group; GP, general practitioner; HF, heart failure; IG, investigational group; inpt, inpatient; IQR, interquartile range; LVEF, left ventricular ejection fraction; NYHA, New York Heart Association functional class; outpt, outpatient; PCP, primary care physician; pt, patient; QOL, quality of life; RCT, randomized controlled trial; RR, risk ratio; Vo_2, oxygen uptake.

Adapted from Lambrinou E, Kalogirou F, Demetris L, et al. Effectiveness of heart failure management programmes with nurse-led discharge planning in reducing re-admissions. A systematic review and meta-analysis. International Journal of Nursing Studies 2012;49:610–24; with permission.

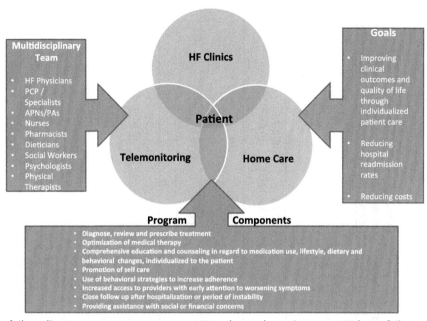

Fig. 1. Heart failure disease management program. APN, advanced practice nurse; HF, heart failure; PA, physician assistant; PCP, primary care practitioner. (*Adapted from* Heart Failure Society of America, Lindenfeld J, Albert NM, et al. HFSA 2010 comprehensive heart failure practice guideline. J Card Fail 2010;16(6):e1–194; with permission.)

care agencies facilitate care, typically with nursing visits, home physical therapy, and social work interventions as necessary. As in clinic models, care team providers undergo specialized HF training. Goals include comprehensive patient and caregiver education on symptom management, self-care strategies, promotion of counseling, and assessment for titration of pharmacotherapy.[43–45] The advantage of this model was that it provides care to HF patients who are frail, immobile, or have significant caregiver or transportation challenges to attending a traditional clinic. Practitioners are able to assess the home environment, identify barriers, and tailor care to achieve realistic and safe goals. A meta-analysis by McAlister and colleagues[23,41] demonstrated that enhancing self-care reduced HF hospitalizations by 34% and all-cause hospitalizations by 20%, but had no effect on mortality. Combination models supporting HF management included telephone follow-up that complemented clinic visits, home visits, and alternating home visits with clinic visits with local practitioners to support medication titration and symptom management.[43] In some home-based programs, researchers reported fewer hospitalizations and days in hospital, in addition to improved quality of life, health care costs, and survival.[23,26,44,46–56]

Structured telephone support (STS) monitoring or self-care management via telephone support involves direct calls to patients. In several meta-

analyses, researchers demonstrated a reduction in HF hospitalizations and all-cause mortality.[38,40] In 2010, a systematic review assessed outcomes in STS (16 studies; n = 5613) and telemonitoring (11 studies; n = 2710), demonstrating a reduction in all-cause mortality for the telemonitoring group with a similar trend in the STS group, though not statistically significant. Reduction in HF hospitalization and cost and an improvement in quality of life were demonstrated with telemonitoring in addition to improvements in patient knowledge, self-care, and functional class.[57]

Many older meta-analyses of outpatient team–based care and HF disease management programs had positive outcomes. In a more recent meta-review of multiple meta-analyses, the investigators stressed the importance of recognizing the complexity and heterogeneity of HF programs. Further evaluation is required to define key characteristics of populations and determine interventions that provide the greatest benefit.[58]

Self-Care Education and Counseling

HF education and counseling is a cornerstone of HF management adherence. Because HF care is performed at home by patients and family or caregivers, a key responsibility of the team is to provide individualized comprehensive education and counseling that promotes self-care (**Table 3**).

Table 2
Selected meta-analyses of heart failure disease management programs

Review	No. of Trials	Total Sampled (N)	Sex (% Males)	Age Range (y)	Professionals	Interventions: 3–4, >4 Type	Intervention Setting No. of Settings Type	All-Cause Mortality	All-Cause Rehospitalization	HF-Related Hospitalization	Quality of Life Pooling (Yes/No = Y/N)
Koshman et al,[70] 2008	12	2060	NR	58–80	MDT, Ph, MD	3–4 Ed, Med, M	4 PDC, H&H, Hm, Outpt, T	OR 0.84 (0.61–1.15)	OR 0.71 (0.54–0.94)	OR 0.69 (0.51–0.94)	N 7/12 studies reported HRQOL +
Clark et al,[38] 2007	14	4264	NR	57–75	MDT	—	1 T, R	RR 0.80 (0.69–0.92)	RR 0.95 (0.89–1.02)	RR 0.79 (0.69–0.89)	—
Gohler et al,[163] 2006	36	8341	37–99	56–79	NL, Ph, MD	3–4 Ed, DC, Med, M	3 Hm, Outpt, T	RD 0.03 (0.01–0.05)	RD 0.08 (0.05–0.11)	NA	—
Jovicic et al,[164] 2006	6	857	53–76	56–76	NL	3–4 Ed, DC, Med, M	3 Hm, Outpt, T	OR 0.93 (0.57–1.51)	OR 0.59 (0.44–0.80)	OR 0.44 (0.27–0.71)	—
Holland,[39] 2005	30	NR	27–99	56–80	NL, MDT	Ed	5 All	RR 0.79 (0.69–0.92)	RR 0.84 (0.79–0.95)	RR 0.70 (0.61–0.81)	—
Kim & Soeken,[165] 2005	4	NR	NR	NR	NL, MDT	3–4 Ed, DC, M	1 PDC, H&H, Hm, Outpt, T	NA	OR 0.87 (0.69–1.04)	NA	—
Phillips et al,[166] 2005	6	949	58	62–79	NL, MDT, MD	3–4 Ed, DC, Med, SS, M	4 PDC, H&H, Hm, Outpt, T	RR 0.80 (0.57–1.13)	RR 0.91 (0.72–1.16)	NA	Y 5/6 studies reported QOL +
Roccaforte et al,[167] 2005	33	3817	42	NR	NL, MDT, Ph, MD	3–4 Ed, DC, Med, M	3 PDC, H&H, Hm, Outpt	OR 0.80 (0.69–0.93)	OR 0.76 (0.69–0.94)	OR 0.58 (0.50–0.67)	N 16/33 studies reported QOL RNPH

Source	No. of studies	No. of patients	Age range	Age		Professionals	No. of components	Components	No. of settings	Settings	RR/OR (95% CI)	RR/OR (95% CI)	RR/OR (95% CI)	HRQOL
Taylor et al,[168] 2005	16	1627	23–86	70–80	—	NL, Card & GP	3–4	Ed, Med, SS, M	4	PDC, H&H, Hm, Outpt, T	OR 0.86 (0.67–1.10)	NA	OR 0.52 (0.39–0.70)	N 8/16 studies reported HRQOL RNPH
Whellan et al,[40] 2005	19	5752	NR	56–80		NL, Card & GP		DC	4	DC, H&H, Hm, Outpt, R	NA	NA	NA	—
Gonseth et al,[169] 2004	54: 27 randomized 27 non randomized	3160	NR	Not summarized		NL, MDT, Ph, MD	>4	Ed, DC, Med, SS	4	PDC, H&H, Hm, Outpt, T	RR 0.75 (0.59–0.96)	RR 0.88 (0.79–0.97)	RR 0.70 (0.62–0.79)	—
Gwadry-Sridhar et al,[170] 2004	8	1239	37–58	71–80.3		MDT		Ed	4	PDC, H&H, Hm, Outpt, T	RR 0.98 (0.72–1.34)	RR 0.79 (0.68–0.91)	NA	N 4/8 studies reported HRQOL RNPH
McAlister et al,[41] 2004	29	5039	NR	56–80		NL, MDT, Ph, Card & GP	>4	Ed, DC, Med, SS, M	4	Hm, Outpt, T, R	RR 0.83 (0.70–0.99)	RR 0.84 (0.75–0.93)	RR 0.73 (0.66–0.82)	—
Phillips et al,[171] 2004	18	3304	62	NR		NL, Ph, MD	3–4	Ed, DC, M	5	All	RR 0.87 (0.73–1.03)	RR 0.75 (0.64–0.88)	RR 0.65 (0.54–0.79)	Y 5/18 studies reported HRQOL +
McAlister et al,[172] 2001	11	2067	NR	63–80		NL, MDT, Card & GP	>4	Ed, DC, Med, SS, M	3	Hm, Outpt, T	RR 0.94 (0.75–1.19)	RR 0.87 (0.79–0.96)	NA	N 5/11 studies reported HRQOL Insufficient data

Professionals: Card &GP, cardiologist and general practitioner MD, cardiologist or general practitioner; MDT, multidisciplinary team; NL, nurse-led; Ph, pharmacist.

Intervention types and settings: DC, support at hospital discharge; Ed, Education; H&H, hospital and home; Hm, home; M, monitoring by home visits or telephone; Med, medication review; Outpt, outpatient clinic; PDC, hospital/predischarge; R, remote provision; SS, social support; T, telephone.

Abbreviations: +, nonsignificant trend favoring intervention; HRQOL, health-related quality of life; NR, not reported; OR, odds ratio; QOL, quality of life; RD, risk difference; RNPH, results not pooled due to heterogeneity; RR, risk ratio.

Adapted from Savard L, Thompson DR, Clark AM. A meta-review of evidence on heart failure disease management programs: the challenges of describing and synthesizing evidence on complex interventions. Trials 2011;12(194):1–10.

Table 3
HF guidelines patient education assessment and components

Patient Education Assessment/ Considerations	Educational Components/Self-care Promotion
Literacy	Cause of heart failure
Cognitive status	Recognition of escalating symptoms with a defined response plan
Psychological state	Indications for medications used and their effects
Culture	Modifying risk factors
Social and financial resources	Dietary recommendations of salt, fluid, and alcohol restrictions
Frequency intensity and duration	Specific activity recommendations
	Understanding importance of treatment with strategies to promote adherence

Adapted from Heart Failure Society of America, Lindenfeld J, Albert NM, et al. HFSA 2010 comprehensive heart failure practice guideline. J Card Fail 2010;16(6):e1–194; with permission.

MULTIDISCIPLINARY TEAM

Given the dynamic demands in the management of HF, a multidisciplinary team, each with their own unique set of skills, may be most effective in executing care for this complex patient population (**Table 4**).

Role of Physicians

Owing to the complex nature of HF, cardiologists specialized in HF typically lead the HF management program, with primary care and other physician specialists collaboratively involved at various stages and in the management of additional disease conditions. Coordinated communication between physicians and specialists is critical to the success of integrated care for the patient.

Role of Nurses

Nurses play an integral role in team management of HF patients. In a physician-directed clinic model, nurses assist with patient management. In a nurse-directed or nurse–managed care model, an initial evaluation of patients is made by cardiologists who determine a treatment plan. Subsequently, nurses, often advanced practice nurses (APNs), have primary responsibility for the management of patients. In this model, nurses may see patients independently or in collaboration with cardiologists as the condition necessitates.[59]

In a study from a physician-directed, nurse-coordinated clinic, outcomes were compared in 134 HF patients before and after referral to the HF program for patients followed for longer than 30 days. After referral, rehospitalizations decreased by 53% and patient's functional status (peak oxygen uptake [Vo$_2$]) and reported quality of life improved.[59,60] In a study of 214 HF patients

referred to an HF program that consisted of cardiologists and HF clinical nurse specialists, there was an 85% reduction in rehospitalizations with estimated cost savings of $9800 per patient, and improved New York Heart Association (NYHA) functional class and peak Vo$_2$ when compared with 6 months before program interventions.[59,61]

In meta-analysis of 18 randomized studies and nonrandomized controlled trials,[15] investigators compared HF clinical care with specialized nurse interventions with usual or conventional care. Clinics had a wide variety of designs and intervention types. Each study included 100 to 500 subjects with nurse interventions focused primarily on patient education and medication optimization, with half of the selected studies incorporating home visits. The investigators concluded that nursing interventions should be an integral part of care provided by HF clinics, as analyses of most studies demonstrated reductions in hospital readmissions or length of stay in the intervention groups. In addition, data suggested that programs involving home visits were more effective than office visits alone, despite being more challenging to use.[15]

Cintron and colleagues,[25] who were pioneers in the formation of specialty HF care managed by nurse practitioners (NPs), demonstrated a 60% reduction in rehospitalizations and an 80% reduction in hospital days after an average 12-month follow-up. In addition, they demonstrated improved patient care satisfaction a 75% net reduction in cost.[59] The influence of program staffing with APNs and physician assistants (PAs) on conforming to GDMT in the outpatient setting was examined in the IMPROVE-HF registry in 14,891 patients. Programmatic staffing with 2 or more APNs or PAs was associated with greater

Table 4
Primary roles and responsibilities of multidisciplinary HF team

Care Team Member	Primary Roles and Responsibility
Physicians	Care team leader Diagnosis Implementation of evidence-based treatment, GDMT Subsequent follow-up aimed at maximizing prognosis and quality of life
Nurses	Reassess the patients' medical and psychosocial needs to tailor interventions and enhance quality of life Implementation of GDMT and risk factor modification Medication titration and adjustment based on reported symptoms or review of diagnostic test results Comprehensive patient/caregiver education regarding knowledge of disease symptom recognition, importance of medications and side effects, lifestyle, and diet changes Self-care promotion
Pharmacists	Resource for clinicians and patients regarding GDMT education and administration Medication reconciliation Monitoring for interactions, contraindications, and potential adverse events of medication regimens
Dieticians	Dietary education, counseling, resources Strategies for patients and caregivers to improve compliance with prescribed dietary recommendations specific to patient
Physical/exercise therapists	Assess and advise patient on reconditioning and training Create an individualized exercise program prescription for improving functional capacity
Social workers/psychologists	Assess impact of illness on quality of life, adjustment to illness and/or hospitalization Identify religious or cultural factors affecting care Address family, grief counseling, or relationship concerns Resource for identifying programs, services or benefits for which a patient may qualify Assist with financial, legal, or insurance issues Assessment of social support or caregiver network Assist with advanced directives and end-of-life discussions
Palliative/advance care planning	Assist with defining goals of care, end-of-life advance care planning, symptom management

Abbreviation: GDMT, guideline-directed medical therapy.
Adapted from Grady KL, Dracup K, Kennedy G, et al. Team management of patients with heart failure. Circulation 2000;102(19):2443–56; with permission.

delivery of HF education and use of ICDs, but equal compliance with use of core HF medications, anticoagulation (atrial fibrillation [AF]), and cardiac resynchronization therapy (CRT).[22]

Role of Pharmacists

Patients with HF are often elderly and may need special consideration with regard to the complexity, challenges, and risks of polypharmacy. Pharmacists can be vigilant gatekeepers to improvements in medication adherence,[50,62–65] reduction in medication errors,[62,64] and positive change in therapeutic outcomes and quality

measures in patient populations that require frequent medication changes and dose adjustment for disease management.[62,66–68] Gattis and colleagues[69] studied the role of a clinical pharmacist intervention within an outpatient HF team. Patients with pharmacist services had fewer nonfatal HF events (9% vs 25%) defined as ED visits or hospitalizations.[62] In 2008, a systematic review found that pharmacist interventions were associated with significant reductions in both all-cause and HF hospitalizations. More pronounced reductions in HF hospitalization rates were observed in multidisciplinary settings in comparison with pharmacist-directed care alone.[68,70]

Role of Dieticians

Lifestyle and dietary restrictions play a key role in the HF treatment plan and patient management. Knowledge and expertise of registered dieticians can assist the HF team and patient to individualize a dietary plan specific to patient needs. Patients with HF and diabetes, chronic kidney disease, dyslipidemia, or other conditions require specialized dietary regimens tailored to the patient's overall nutritional requirements.[23] In research, investigators identified the beneficial role of dieticians in the HF team.[26,43] In a 2005 study, when patients with HF were randomized to a dietician education group on a 2 g/d dietary sodium prescription versus usual care, intervention patients had a significant decrease in sodium intake at 3 months.[71]

Role of Exercise/Physical Therapists

Patients with HF are often deconditioned from inactivity related to the burden of HF symptoms, fear of worsening symptoms, recurrent hospitalizations, lack of motivation, depressive symptoms, or limitations related to other comorbidities.

Exercise training in patients with HF is safe and with potential physiologic benefits, can improve survival, exercise capacity, functional status, and quality of life, and can reduce the risk of hospitalizations.[23,72–74] The largest multicenter, randomized controlled trial, HF-ACTION (Heart Failure: A Controlled Trial Investigating Outcomes of Exercise Training), enrolled 2331 medically stable HF outpatients who were randomly assigned to usual care plus aerobic exercise training or to usual care alone. Exercise training resulted in insignificant reductions of all-cause mortality or hospitalization; however, after adjustment for highly prognostic predictors, exercise training was associated with modest but significant reductions in all-cause mortality or hospitalization and cardiovascular mortality or cardiovascular hospitalization. Exercise training was also associated with modest but statistically significant improvements in self-reported health status at 3 months, and persisted over time.[23,72,73]

The strength of evidence led the Centers for Medicare and Medicaid Services to expand coverage for cardiac rehabilitation services to patients with stable, chronic HF meeting specified criteria.[74]

Guideline-directed exercise recommendations are for appropriately selected patients with HF to increase exercise intensity and duration in a supervised setting, with a goal of 30 minutes per day, 5 days per week.[23] Cardiac rehabilitation with an exercise prescription includes intensity, frequency, duration, progression, behavioral and lifestyle risk factor reduction, health education, and personal counseling.[74]

Role of Social Workers and Psychologists

The diagnosis, prognosis, symptom progression, uncertain illness trajectory, and frequent exacerbations of HF can be overwhelming and may provoke stress, anxiety, and depression. Consequently, patients may be unable to comprehend or adhere to a treatment plan, resulting in poor self-management. Psychologists and social workers help patients and family members cope with the psychosocial effects of HF. Several studies have examined the effectiveness of psychosocial interventions in patients with cardiac disease. A Cochrane review concluded that although psychological interventions showed no effect on total or cardiac mortality, small reductions in anxiety and depression were found in patients with coronary heart disease.[75,76] In a meta-analysis of psychological treatment of cardiac patients, researchers concluded that treatment reduced mortality in men, in addition to usual care.[77] Patients starting psychological treatment 2 months after a cardiac event showed an impressive mortality reduction of 72% in the first 2 years. In another report, Child and colleagues[76] found a reduction in the percentage of patients reporting depression and anxiety (13% and 19%) following a program that offers a range of therapy treatment interventions.

OUTPATIENT MONITORING AND MANAGEMENT SYSTEMS
How to Detect Congestion

Evidence of congestion is a leading cause for decompensation and hospitalization for patients with HF.[78] Several technologies or monitoring programs designed to detect volume overload at an early stage and prevent exacerbation of symptoms that lead to disease progression, hospitalization, or increased mortality have been studied.

Telemonitoring

Telemonitoring uses a variety of devices to collect data from patients and transmit them to a health care provider via telephone, Internet, or wireless technology. Data may include weight, blood pressure, heart rate (HR), electrocardiogram tracings, or questions related to HF symptoms such as shortness of breath or fatigue. In ambulatory HF, 2 meta-analyses showed that telemonitoring improved mortality and reduced hospitalizations at 6 to 12 months of follow-up.[79,80]

The large, randomized Tele-HF (Telemonitoring to Improve Heart Failure Outcomes)[81] and TIM-HF (Telemedical Interventional Monitoring in Heart Failure)[82] studies found no significant differences between telemonitoring and usual care groups. Although more research is needed, their findings may be due to underuse of the therapy. Fourteen percent of subjects randomized to telemonitoring in the Tele-HF study did not use it, and at the end of study only 55% of patients were still using the system a minimum of 3 days per week.[81] Telemonitoring may be useful when adherence to schedules and instructions are maintained and health care provider follow-up is optimized.

Cardiac Device Monitoring

A CRT defibrillator (CRT-D) device in patients with left ventricular ejection fraction (LVEF) of 35% or less and stage C HF is a Class 1A recommendation if all criteria for use are met.[83] Cardiac devices implanted for primary prevention of sudden cardiac death and cardiac resynchronization also provide other parameters that may identify patients at risk for HF deterioration. In a retrospective analysis of 4 studies (PARTNERS-HF, OFISSER, FAST, and CONNECT), Whellan and colleagues[84] sought to identify patients with CRT-D devices at risk of early HF readmission. Patients were monitored monthly for high AF burden, rapid ventricular rate (RVR) during AF, high fluid index ($\geq$60), low activity levels, abnormal autonomic function (high HR at night or low HR variability), and device therapy issues (low CRT pacing or ICD shocks). Daily impedance, high AF burden with RVR greater than 90 beats/min, decreased CRT-D pacing (<90%), and mean HR at night greater than 80 beats/min were significant predictors of 30-day HF readmission when patients exhibited 3 or more parameters in the highest risk category. Patients who exhibited any 2 high-risk parameters or had a very high fluid index ($\geq$100) had a 5.5-fold increase in hospitalization with pulmonary congestion within the next month. Intrathoracic impedance measurement detects pulmonary congestion and may be useful for monitoring pulmonary fluid status. The proposed threshold for an impedance alert of 60 Ω per day is sensitive but not specific for assessment of HF; further adjustment of threshold settings may define an optimal balance between sensitivity and specificity.[85]

Implantable Hemodynamic Monitoring

A new era has begun in the management of NYHA class III HF patients. The CardioMEMS Heart Failure System is the first and only device approved (as of May 28, 2014) by the Food and Drug Administration (FDA) that measures pulmonary artery pressure. This miniature, fully implantable, wireless pulmonary artery pressure monitoring system was studied in the CHAMPION trial for use in HF from any cause or ejection fraction, NYHA class III patients, who had an HF hospitalization in the past 12 months. In this trial, pulmonary artery monitoring significantly reduced HF-related hospital admissions by 37% at 15 months and improved the quality of life of patients.[86] Results were more impressive among patients with HF with preserved ejection fraction (HFpEF) by reducing hospitalization by 50% at 6 months and 60% at 5 months in comparison with the control group.[87] Hemodynamic data obtained from the system should be used in addition to weights, symptoms, laboratory values, and other traditional markers of volume excess and functional decline. The CardioMEMS is contraindicated in patients unable to take dual antiplatelet therapy or anticoagulants for 1 month after implantation.

Use of Evidence-Based Therapies

Despite improving national trends, a gap remains between GDMT recommendations and actual clinical practice. Performance measures were established to address this gap, but these measures may be insufficient to improve postdischarge outcomes of such a complex medical condition.[88–90] It is well established that patients with HF with reduced ejection fraction (HFrEF) should receive recommended doses of β-blockers,[91–93] angiotensin-converting enzyme (ACE) inhibitors/angiotensin receptor blockers (ARBs),[94–98] and aldosterone antagonists.[96,99–101] Despite this, less than one-third of eligible patients hospitalized with HF received aldosterone antagonists,[102] although this may be related to renal function and serum potassium level. In the OPTIMIZE-HF registry, adherence to guideline-directed therapies resulted in shorter length of stay and reduced readmissions.[1,102,103] Hydralazine and nitrate therapy is recommended for African Americans with HFrEF in addition to standard GDMT.[1,104–107] Guideline-directed medical therapies are also highly cost effective. In a study examining the incremental cost-effectiveness ratios of ACE inhibitors, β-blockers, and aldosterone antagonists, the greatest gains in quality-adjusted life-years occurred when all 3 guideline-directed therapies were provided.[2,83] However, despite accounting for roughly half of the HF population, there remain limited data regarding efficacious therapies for HFpEF patients.

Digoxin, which has hemodynamic, neurohormonal, and electrophysiologic effects, may be beneficial in HF.[103,108,109] Recent reanalysis of the Digitalis Investigation Group Trial demonstrated that digoxin reduced 30-day all-cause hospital admissions in ambulatory older patients with chronic systolic HF.[103,110,111] In addition, Medicare beneficiaries receiving a discharge prescription for digoxin did not have higher mortality at 1 year.[1,112] However, a reduction in 30-day all-cause hospital admissions was not demonstrated in older patients with chronic HFpEF (LVEF >45%).[103,110,113] Further study of digoxin is warranted, as the effects of digoxin in a contemporary sample and its effects on readmissions have not been examined.

A promising new therapy is the angiotensin receptor neprilysin inhibitor, LCZ696. This therapy was compared with enalapril in a double-blind randomized controlled trial, PARADIGM-HF. The trial was stopped early, after a median follow-up of 27 months, because the margin for an overwhelming benefit for LCZ696 had been crossed. LCZ696 was shown to be superior to enalapril in reducing the risks of death and HF hospitalizations.[103,114]

Optimization of Medications

Optimization of HF therapies is critical. Clinical status should be continuously reassessed, with every attempt made to reach target doses of ACE inhibitors/ARBs, β-blockers, and aldosterone antagonists[103,115] used in clinical trials, if clinically indicated. It should not be assumed that smaller doses are as effective, as this has not been studied. Often these medication titrations can be made not only through clinical visits but also through other forms of direct communication. The use of GDMT at optimal doses has been shown to improve mortality, reduce readmissions, and result in cost savings.[2,116,117]

Fluid Management

Preventing clinical and subclinical congestion is critical to reducing rehospitalization rates.[5,118] Sodium restriction is also important in the postdischarge period to control fluid management.[83] Loop diuretic therapy is a mainstay of congestion management, as novel therapies such as vasopressin antagonists, adenosine-blocking agents, and ultrafiltration yielded mixed results.[2,7] Diuretic therapy may worsen renal function during hospitalization; however, it is generally transient, does not represent kidney injury, and should not prevent aggressive diuresis.[5,8] ACE inhibitors or ARBs also may transiently worsen renal function, despite demonstrating mortality benefits, and should be used if appropriate.[7,10]

During hospitalization, most patients will have significant improvement in clinical congestion, but may have persistent subclinical congestion. Elevated natriuretic peptide levels are a poor prognostic feature at the time of discharge and may warrant further evaluation.[8,88] Initial and maintenance diuretic dosing should be guided by blood pressure measurement (supine and orthostatic) and renal function.[10,91] Metolazone may be used as adjunctive therapy when patients are unresponsive to loop diuretic therapy, but carries a significant risk of hyponatremia, hyperkalemia, other electrolyte abnormalities and hypovolemia. Aldosterone antagonists may be beneficial in reducing congestion, and have been demonstrated to significantly reduce early hospitalization rates.[88,89,94,96]

Tolvaptan, a vasopressin antagonist, may be helpful in patients with hyponatremia, relative hypotension, or impaired renal function; however, long-term effects on hospitalization have been neutral, and efficacy in patients with hyponatremia requires further study.[91,92,99,100] Furthermore, tolvaptan requires hospital admission for initiation and may be costly.

PALLIATIVE CARE

As the chronicity of HF ensues, it is imperative that patients be made aware of care options throughout the progression of their illness. Palliative care is interdisciplinary care that is offered simultaneously with medical therapies. Palliative care focuses on improving quality of life while ensuring symptom relief and interventions that address psychological, emotional, physical, and spiritual needs.[1,94–96,103] Palliative care has been associated with symptom control, reduced hospitalizations, increased patient and caregiver satisfaction, and decreased costs in patients with HF.[1,96,99,104,106,107] Furthermore, palliative and supportive care potentially improves the quality of life in patients with symptomatic HF (Class I, 2013 American College of Cardiology [ACCF]/AHA guidelines).[83]

The process of shared decision making is a key principle of palliative care. Patients and clinicians should have discussions to determine values, preferences, and goals about symptom relief, pain control, life-prolonging therapies, and end-of-life care.[103,110] By strengthening communication between health care professionals, patients, and their caregivers, palliative care helps facilitate treatment plans matching the values and goals of patients.[1,103,108,109]

The optimal time to discuss patient preferences and shared decision making is in the ambulatory setting, preferably with an HF team.[103,110,111] When the patient is hospitalized, a more emergent situation evolves; this should be a time to review decisions, rather than to introduce advanced care decisions.[103,110,113] In past studies, there were often substantial differences between patient preferences, and the understanding of these preferences by the physician and their families. This point emphasizes the need to explore care preferences from the primary source, the patient, whenever possible.[103,114,116,117] Furthermore, clinicians need to understand that for some patients, priorities may not be on life-prolonging measures[103,115,118]; greater importance may be on symptom relief and quality of life.[2,103,116,117,119,120]

ADVANCE CARE PLANNING
Outpatient Intravenous Diuresis

There still remains a large group of patients with refractory HF symptoms despite optimal medical therapy that includes diuretic therapies.[91,121] Limited options exist for outpatients who remain fluid overloaded. Therapies for end-stage (stage D) HF patients should be directed toward symptom control, improvement in quality of life, rehospitalization reduction, and defining end-of-life goals.[83,122,123]

Outpatient intravenous (IV) diuretics can be used as palliative support for stage C or D refractory patients to relieve congestive symptoms. Minimal data are available regarding outpatient IV diuresis[121,124] and are limited to mainly small retrospective or nonrandomized studies. Safety of outpatient IV diuresis has been demonstrated, and in some study participants it decreased congestive symptoms, increased fluid weight loss, and improved NYHA class.[125–129] In addition, HF hospitalization was reduced. Ryder and colleagues[126] found that 72% of patients were stabilized and did not require hospitalization,[124] and Banerjee and colleagues[129] noted that 94% of patients were not admitted within 28 days following their outpatient IV diuresis regimen.[126–128] Unsurprisingly, considerable cost savings were noted when hospitalization was not required.[126,127,129]

Further benefit was seen when outpatients receiving IV diuretics were linked with an HF disease management program.[124,126,127,129] Patients at high risk for recurrent HF exacerbation were closely monitored and able to receive an immediate response to changes in clinical status. An essential component of IV diuretic programs is frequent patient reassessment by HF specialists within days following outpatient IV diuresis to determine overall response and the need for diuretic adjustment.[126,127,129]

Inotropes

Approximately 5% of the HF population is considered end-stage (stage D), or having refractory symptoms despite maximal medical therapy.[124,126,127,130,131] Many stage D patients are hospitalized with an acute exacerbation of symptoms. In a global survey of 666 hospitals, 39% of all hospital admissions for acute HF used inotropic therapies.[126,127,132,133] Positive inotropic therapy is indicated to stabilize a patient in acute or chronic hemodynamically compromised states as a bridge to transplant or mechanical support or as a bridge to a decision.[130,131,134,135]

Some patients remain inotrope dependent and cannot safely be weaned without experiencing hypoperfusion, symptomatic hypotension, or worsening symptoms.[132,133,135] However, patients may be stable enough to be discharged home on IV inotropes; and some can be weaned from support before transplant.[133–135] When advanced surgery is not an option, maintenance on IV inotropes may be the only way to allow patients to be discharged to home.[135,136] Conservatively, there are 6200 to 8800 patients nationally receiving home inotropic therapy, and the coordination of the care of these patients ideally is delivered through a team-based approach including home nursing.[134,137]

The use of inotropic agents and the options available (oral and IV, intermittent and continuous, short-term and long-term) have been studied retrospectively and prospectively in ambulatory patients. Most commonly studied has been the β-adrenergic agonist dobutamine and the phosphodiesterase inhibitors milrinone and enoximone. Several studies reported an association between oral inotropes and higher mortality rates when used chronically in ambulatory HF patients,[133,135,138–141] and were not approved by the FDA. Intermittent use of home inotropes was practiced in the past, but no placebo-controlled studies documented survival benefits, and this option is no longer supported in the ACCF/AHA guidelines.[83,133,137] Despite the increased mortality seen in a few randomized controlled studies with home dobutamine,[133,138–143] continuous home inotropic therapy is used today as palliative care to relieve symptoms or as a bridge to transplant.[83,131,133]

Most studies on home inotropic support were retrospective, in a small number of patients awaiting heart transplantation. Several studies reported an improvement in hemodynamics, symptoms, or functional status of patients when on home inotropes.[142–146] A prospective study of 21 patients awaiting transplant at home on IV inotropes reported a decrease in the number of hospitalizations compared with pre-inotrope treatment.[147] In other studies, hospital rates and length of hospital stay were decreased in patients on home inotropes,[144–146,148–150] and health care costs were considerably less when patients received IV inotropes at home rather than in a hospital setting.[147,149] Among the studies, mortality rates varied considerably. In a retrospective study of patients discharged to home on either dobutamine or milrinone, there were no mortality differences by IV therapy.[148–151] However, increased length of time on home inotropes was associated with worse outcomes. Patients receiving home milrinone therapy for less than 3 months had better survival rates to transplant compared with patients on longer duration of therapy.[147,149,152] In a small study of stage D inotrope-dependent patients discharged to home and not on an active transplant list, 6-month survival was only 26%.[136,151] In a larger retrospective Medicare analysis of 331 patients receiving dobutamine, milrinone, or both, mortality was greater than 40% at 6 months.[150,152]

With the increased mortality rates seen with IV inotropes, the 2013 ACCF/AHA guidelines state that long-term use of continuous inotropes in the absence of specific indications was potentially harmful, or a IIb indication. Continuous IV inotrope use is reasonable as a bridge to standard medical therapy, mechanical circulatory support, or transplant; alternatively it may be considered palliative therapy for symptom control in selected patients with stage D HF.[83,136] Patients and families must be fully informed that improved symptom control comes with additional risks, and long-term IV inotrope use may ultimately be harmful.[136,137]

Thus, the decision to send patients home on inotropes should be made only after aggressive attempts of inotrope weaning and optimal titration of oral medical therapy.[136,150] If patients are inotrope dependent and are to be discharged to home, the decision should be guided by the goal of symptom relief and patient preference.[83,103,135]

MECHANICAL CIRCULATORY SUPPORT

When medical options have failed, an evaluation for MCS may be offered to control symptoms and improve the quality of life and survival.[1,110,153–155] Ideally, discussions of advance care planning along with the possibility of MCS should be done in an outpatient, nonemergent setting, where patients actively participate in decision-making processes.[103,110,154] Partnering with the MCS team, palliative care can help meet the needs of patients and their families, and set expectations of care, and should be offered to all patients during the time of MCS evaluation.[1,110,155]

Mechanical circulatory devices have been increasingly used not only as a bridge to transplant[103,110,156] but also for long-term destination therapy (DT) support with continuous-flow left ventricular assist devices (LVADs), after their approval in 2010.[1,157] Using INTERMACS data, the indication for more than 40% of implanted LVADs between 2011 and 2013 were as DT.[156,158] The combination of increasing numbers with end-stage HF, stagnant donor heart availability, and continued improvements in MCS may equate to an increase in the number of patients living with these devices.[1,157]

To enhance independence with MCS, discharging patients to home becomes an important consideration for patients and families, in addition to the health care institutions bearing the costs of ventricular assist device (VAD)-related hospitalizations.[4,158] Many centers have been reluctant to discharge patients with biventricular assist devices (BiVADs) owing to the question of safety concerns and perception of increased adverse events. However, Thomas and colleagues[4] reported a BiVAD discharge rate of almost 60%, with similar outcomes on readmissions and survival data at 6 months and 1 year compared with LVAD patients discharged to home.[3] Similarly, Creaser and colleagues[159] reported 58% of BiVADs successfully discharged to home, with 93% successfully bridged to transplant.[3] Patients implanted with the total artificial heart (TAH) were also successfully discharged to home,[6,156,160,161] with one program reporting a 44% discharge rate. Of those discharged to home, 87% of TAH support time was out of the hospital, with 100% of outpatients proceeding to transplant.[9,156]

There are considerable benefits to MCS patients when discharged to home. LVAD patients reported improvements in quality of life and demonstrated greater functional ability in movement, mobility, and ambulation following hospital discharge.[11,162] Discharging BiVAD patients home allows time to physically rehabilitate from the surgical experience, achieve medical stability, and improve overall nutrition and strength before proceeding to transplant surgery.[89,90,159] In addition, TAH patients reported improvements in quality of life with discharge to home and remained ambulatory.[92,93,161]

For MCS patients eligible to be discharged from the hospital, close monitoring and follow-up is needed in an ambulatory care setting for long-term HF management. MCS patients are complex, and require a multidisciplinary HF and VAD team approach to successfully maintain medical and hemodynamic stability over time. Key aspects of outpatient integrated care include home health nursing visits, frequent laboratory monitoring, regular outpatient clinical assessments from cardiologists, APNs and VAD nurse coordinators, and support from community providers.[4,95,97,98,159]

SUMMARY AND FUTURE DIRECTIONS

Management of HF requires an extensive team-based multidisciplinary effort. Such an approach includes coordination with patients and their family/caregivers to ensure optimization of GDMT (including devices), frequent and regular assessment of volume status, ongoing HF education, use of cardiac rehabilitation, continued assessment for use of advanced therapies, and advance care planning. Complex management often involves a village of specialists (HF cardiologist, APN, general cardiologist, pharmacist, dietician, social worker, and numerous others). It is important to recognize that the most critical member of this team is the patient, as achieving success with HF is not possible without the active engagement of the patient and family/caregivers. Although optimal implementation of GDMT can achieve amelioration of clinical HF, reduce hospitalizations, and reduce mortality, not all patients respond. New therapies may provide incremental benefit (ie, LCZ686), as have advances in monitoring technology (ie, CardioMEMS). Additional future mechanisms may include systems such as mobile applications to aid medication compliance or monitor exercise. New interventions will have to balance ease of use, effectiveness, and cost. Ultimately, team-based approaches for HF, combining the strategies outlined in this article tailored to the individual dynamics and preferences of patients, may lead to further improvements in reducing hospitalizations, improving the quality of life, decreasing mortality, and providing enhanced value.

REFERENCES

1. Goldstein NE, May CW, Meier DE. Comprehensive care for mechanical circulatory support: a new frontier for synergy with palliative care. Circ Heart Fail 2011;4(4):519–27.
2. Banka G, Heidenreich PA, Fonarow GC. Incremental cost-effectiveness of guideline-directed medical therapies for heart failure. J Am Coll Cardiol 2013; 61(13):1440–6.
3. Go AS, Mozaffarian D, Roger VL, et al. Heart disease and stroke statistics—2014 update. Circulation 2014;129(3):e28–292.
4. Thomas SS, Smallwood J, Smith CM, et al. Discharge outcomes in patients with paracorporeal biventricular assist devices. Ann Thorac Surg 2014;97(3):894–900.
5. Gheorghiade M, Follath F, Ponikowski P, et al. Assessing and grading congestion in acute heart failure: a scientific statement from the acute heart failure committee of the heart failure association of the European Society of Cardiology and endorsed by the European Society of Intensive Care Medicine. Eur J Heart Fail 2010;12(5):423–33.
6. Braunschweig F, Cowie MR, Auricchio A. What are the costs of heart failure? Europace 2011;13(Suppl 2):ii13–7.
7. Goldsmith SR, Brandimarte F, Gheorghiade M. Congestion as a therapeutic target in acute heart failure syndromes. Prog Cardiovasc Dis 2010; 52(5):383–92.
8. Blair JE, Pang PS, Schrier RW, et al. Changes in renal function during hospitalization and soon after discharge in patients admitted for worsening heart failure in the placebo group of the EVEREST trial. Eur Heart J 2011;32(20):2563–72.
9. Kim SM, Han HR. Evidence-based strategies to reduce readmission in patients with heart failure. J Nurse Pract 2013;9.
10. Valika AA, Gheorghiade M. ACE inhibitor therapy for heart failure in patients with impaired renal function: a review of the literature. Heart Fail Rev 2013; 18:135–40.
11. Stewart S. Heart failure management—a team based approach. Aust Fam Physician 2010; 39(12):894–6.
12. Vinson JM, Rich MW, Sperry JC, et al. Early readmission of elderly patients with congestive heart failure. J Am Geriatr Soc 1990;38(12):1290–5.
13. Michalsen A, König G, Thimme W. Preventable causative factors leading to hospital admission with decompensated heart failure. Heart 1998; 80(5):437–41.
14. Tsuyuki RT, McKelvie RS, Arnold JM, et al. Acute precipitants of congestive heart failure exacerbations. Arch Intern Med 2001;161(19): 2337–42.
15. Gustafsson F, Arnold JM. Heart failure clinics and outpatient management: review of the evidence and call for quality assurance. Eur Heart J 2004; 25(18):1596–604.
16. Wagner EH. The role of patient care teams in chronic disease management. BMJ 2000; 320(7234):569.
17. Institute of Medicine (US), Olsen L, Saunders RS, et al. Patients charting the course. Wahington DC: National Academies Press; 2011. p. 187–212.

18. Hauptman PJ, Rich MW, Heidenreich PA, et al. The heart failure clinic: a consensus statement of the Heart Failure Society of America. J Card Fail 2008;14:801–15.

19. Bernard S. Disease management: a pharmaceutical industry perspective. Pharmaceutical Exec 1995;15:48–50.

20. DePasquale EC, Fonarow GC. A practical guide for reducing readmissions in heart failure. In: Maisel A, Filippatos G, editors. Heart failure: the expert's approach. Delhi: Jaypee Brothers Medical Publishers; 2014. p. 183–92.

21. Krumholz HM, Currie PM, Riegel B, et al. A taxonomy for disease management: a scientific statement from the American Heart Association Disease Management Taxonomy Writing Group. Circulation 2006;114(13):1432–45.

22. Albert NM, Fonarow GC, Yancy CW, et al. Outpatient cardiology practices with advanced practice nurses and physician assistants provide similar delivery of recommended therapies (findings from IMPROVE HF). Am J Cardiol 2010;105(12):1773–9.

23. Heart Failure Society of America, Lindenfeld J, Albert NM, et al. HFSA 2010 comprehensive heart failure practice guideline. J Card Fail 2010;16(6):e1–194.

24. Adams KF, Lindenfeld J, Arnold J, et al. HFSA 2006 comprehensive heart failure practice guideline. J Card Fail 2006;12:e1–119.

25. Cintron G, Bigas C, Linares E, et al. Nurse practitioner role in a chronic congestive heart failure clinic: in-hospital time, costs, and patient satisfaction. Heart Lung 1983;12(3):237–40.

26. Rich MW, Beckham V, Wittenberg C, et al. A multidisciplinary intervention to prevent the readmission of elderly patients with congestive heart failure. N Engl J Med 1995;333(18):1190–5.

27. Rich MW, Vinson JM, Sperry JC, et al. Prevention of readmission in elderly patients with congestive heart failure: results of a prospective, randomized pilot study. J Gen Intern Med 1993;8(11):585–90.

28. Howlett JG. Specialist heart failure clinics must evolve to stay relevant. Can J Cardiol 2014;30(3):276–80.

29. Lasater M. The effect of a nurse-managed CHF clinic on patient readmission and length of stay. Home Healthc Nurse 1996;14(5):351–6.

30. Smith LE, Fabbri SA, Pai R, et al. Symptomatic improvement and reduced hospitalization for patients attending a cardiomyopathy clinic. Clin Cardiol 1997;20(11):949–54.

31. Cline C, Israelsson B, Willenheimer RB, et al. Cost effective management programme for heart failure reduces hospitalisation. Heart 1998;80(5):442–6.

32. Dahl J, Penque S. The effects of an advanced practice nurse-directed heart failure program. Nurse Pract 2000;25(3):61–2, 65–8, 71–4 passim.

33. McDonald K, Ledwidge M, Cahill J, et al. Heart failure management: multidisciplinary care has intrinsic benefit above the optimization of medical care. J Card Fail 2002;8(3):142–8.

34. Atienza F, Anguita M, Martinez-Alzamora N, et al. Multicenter randomized trial of a comprehensive hospital discharge and outpatient heart failure management program. Eur J Heart Fail 2004;6(5):643–52.

35. Thompson DR, Roebuck A, Stewart S. Effects of a nurse-led, clinic and home-based intervention on recurrent hospital use in chronic heart failure. Eur J Heart Fail 2005;7(3):377–84.

36. Del Sindaco D, Pulignano G, Minardi G, et al. Two-year outcome of a prospective, controlled study of a disease management programme for elderly patients with heart failure. J Cardiovasc Med 2007;8(5):324–9.

37. Jaarsma T, van der Wal MH, Lesman-Leegte I, et al. Effect of moderate or intensive disease management program on outcome in patients with heart failure. Arch Intern Med 2008;168(3):316–24.

38. Clark RA, Inglis SC, McAlister FA, et al. Telemonitoring or structured telephone support programmes for patients with chronic heart failure: systematic review and meta-analysis. BMJ 2007;334(7600):942.

39. Holland R. Systematic review of multidisciplinary interventions in heart failure. Heart 2005;91(7):899–906.

40. Whellan DJ, Hasselblad V, Peterson E, et al. Meta-analysis and review of heart failure disease management randomized controlled clinical trials. Am Heart J 2005;149(4):722–9.

41. McAlister FA, Stewart S, Ferrua S, et al. Multidisciplinary strategies for the management of heart failure patients at high risk for admission: a systematic review of randomized trials. J Am Coll Cardiol 2004;44(4):810–9.

42. Andrikopoulou E, Abbate K, Whellan DJ. Conceptual model for heart failure disease management. Can J Cardiol 2014;30(3):304–11.

43. Jaarsma T. Inter-professional team approach to patients with heart failure. Heart 2005;91(6):832–8.

44. Stewart S, Horowitz JD. Home-based intervention in congestive heart failure: long-term implications on readmission and survival. Circulation 2002;105(24):2861–6.

45. Doughty RN, Wright SP, Pearl A, et al. Randomized, controlled trial of integrated heart failure management: the Auckland Heart Failure Management Study. Eur Heart J 2002;23(2):139–46.

46. Riegel B, Carlson B, Glaser D, et al. Which patients with heart failure respond best to multidisciplinary disease management? J Card Fail 2000;6(4):290–9.

47. Blue L, Lang E, McMurray JJ, et al. Randomised controlled trial of specialist nurse intervention in heart failure. BMJ 2001;323(7315):715–8.

48. Jaarsma T, Halfens R, Abu-Saad H, et al. Effects of education and support on self-care and resource utilization in patients with heart failure. Eur Heart J 1999;20(9):673–82.

49. Kasper EK, Gerstenblith G, Hefter G, et al. A randomized trial of the efficacy of multidisciplinary care in heart failure outpatients at high risk of hospital readmission. J Am Coll Cardiol 2002;39(3):471–80.

50. Stewart S, Pearson S, Horowitz JD. Effects of a home-based intervention among patients with congestive heart failure discharged from acute hospital care. Arch Intern Med 1998;158(10): 1067–72.

51. Stewart S, Marley JE, Horowitz JD. Effects of a multidisciplinary, home-based intervention on planned readmissions and survival among patients with chronic congestive heart failure: a randomised controlled study. Lancet 1999;354(9184): 1077–83.

52. Stewart S, Vandenbroek AJ, Pearson S, et al. Prolonged beneficial effects of a home-based intervention on unplanned readmissions and mortality among patients with congestive heart failure. Arch Intern Med 1999;159(3):257–61.

53. Riegel B, Carlson B, Kopp Z, et al. Effect of a standardized nurse case-management telephone intervention on resource use in patients with chronic heart failure. Arch Intern Med 2002;162(6):705–12.

54. Laramee AS, Levinsky SK, Sargent J, et al. Case management in a heterogeneous congestive heart failure population—a randomized controlled trial. Arch Intern Med 2003;163(7):809–17.

55. Naylor MD, Brooten DA, Campbell RL, et al. Transitional care of older adults hospitalized with heart failure: a randomized, controlled trial. J Am Geriatr Soc 2004;52(5):675–84.

56. Anderson C, Deepak BV, Amoateng-Adjepong Y, et al. Benefits of comprehensive inpatient education and discharge planning combined with outpatient support in elderly patients with congestive heart failure. Congest Heart Fail 2005;11(6): 315–21.

57. Inglis SC, Clark RA, McAlister FA, et al. Which components of heart failure programmes are effective? A systematic review and meta-analysis of the outcomes of structured telephone support or telemonitoring as the primary component of chronic heart failure management in 8323 patients: abridged Cochrane review. Eur J Heart Fail 2011; 13(9):1028–40.

58. Savard LA, Thompson DR, Clark AM. A meta-review of evidence on heart failure disease management programs: the challenges of describing and synthesizing evidence on complex interventions. Trials 2011;12:194.

59. Grady KL, Dracup K, Kennedy G, et al. Team management of patients with heart failure: a statement for healthcare professionals from The Cardiovascular Nursing Council of the American Heart Association. Circulation 2000;102(19):2443–56.

60. Hanumanthu S, Butler J, Chomsky D, et al. Effect of a heart failure program on hospitalization frequency and exercise tolerance. Circulation 1997; 96(9):2842–8.

61. Fonarow GC, Stevenson LW, Walden JA, et al. Impact of a comprehensive heart failure management program on hospital readmission and functional status of patients with advanced heart failure. J Am Coll Cardiol 1997;30(3):725–32.

62. Milfred-Laforest SK, Chow SL, Didomenico RJ, et al. Clinical pharmacy services in heart failure: an opinion paper from the Heart Failure Society of America and American College of Clinical Pharmacy Cardiology Practice and Research Network. J Card Fail 2013;19(5):354–69.

63. Eggink RN, Lenderink AW, Widdershoven JW, et al. The effect of a clinical pharmacist discharge service on medication discrepancies in patients with heart failure. Pharm World Sci 2010;32(6): 759–66.

64. LaForest S, Gee J, Pugacz A, et al. SERIOUS medication reconciliation clinic: improving transitions of care. J Card Fail 2010;16:112m.

65. Murray MD, Young J, Hoke S, et al. Pharmacist intervention to improve medication adherence in heart failure: a randomized trial. Ann Intern Med 2007;146(10):714–25.

66. Rodgers JE, Stough WG. Underutilization of evidence-based therapies in heart failure: the pharmacist's role. Pharmacotherapy 2007;27(4 Pt 2): 18S–28S.

67. Campbell PT, Tremaglio J, Bhardwaj A, et al. Utility of daily diuretic orders for identifying acute decompensated heart failure patients for quality improvement. Crit Pathw Cardiol 2010;9(3):148–51.

68. Cheng JW, Cooke-Ariel H. Pharmacists' role in the care of patients with heart failure: review and future evolution. J Manag Care Pharm 2014;20(2): 206–13.

69. Gattis WA, Hasselblad V, Whellan DJ, et al. Reduction in heart failure events by the addition of a clinical pharmacist to the heart failure management team: results of the Pharmacist in Heart Failure Assessment Recommendation and Monitoring (PHARM) Study. Arch Intern Med 1999;159(16): 1939–45.

70. Koshman SL, Charrois TL, Simpson SH, et al. Pharmacist care of patients with heart failure: a systematic review of randomized trials. Arch Intern Med 2008;168(7):687–94.

71. Arcand JA, Brazel S, Joliffe C, et al. Education by a dietitian in patients with heart failure results in improved adherence with a sodium-restricted diet: a randomized trial. Am Heart J 2005; 150(4):716.

72. O'Connor CM, Whellan DJ, Lee KL, et al. Efficacy and safety of exercise training in patients with chronic heart failure: HF-ACTION randomized controlled trial. JAMA 2009;301(14):1439–50.

73. Flynn KE, Piña IL, Whellan DJ, et al. Effects of exercise training on health status in patients with chronic heart failure: HF-ACTION randomized controlled trial. JAMA 2009;301(14):1451–9.

74. Decision Memo for Cardiac Rehabilitation (CR) Programs—Chronic heart failure (CAG-00437N). cmsgov. Available at: http://www.cms.gov/medicare-coverage-database/details/nca-decision-memo.aspx?NCAId=270. Accessed November 11, 2014.

75. Rees K, Bennett P, West R, et al. Psychological interventions for coronary heart disease. Cochrane Database Syst Rev 2004;(2):CD002902.

76. Child A, Sanders J, Sigel P, et al. Meeting the psychological needs of cardiac patients: an integrated stepped-care approach within a cardiac rehabilitation setting. Br J Cardiol 2010;17.

77. Linden W, Phillips MJ, Leclerc J. Psychological treatment of cardiac patients: a meta-analysis. Eur Heart J 2007;28(24):2972–84.

78. Fonarow GC, Abraham WT, Albert NM, et al. Factors identified as precipitating hospital admissions for heart failure and clinical outcomes: findings from OPTIMIZE-HF. Arch Intern Med 2008; 168(8):847–54.

79. Klersy C, De Silvestri A, Gabutti G, et al. A meta-analysis of remote monitoring of heart failure patients. J Am Coll Cardiol 2009;54(18):1683–94.

80. Inglis SC, Clark RA, McAlister FA, et al. Structured telephone support or telemonitoring programmes for patients with chronic heart failure. Cochrane Database Syst Rev 2010;(8):CD007228. Inglis SC, editor.

81. Chaudhry SI, Mattera JA, Curtis JP, et al. Telemonitoring in patients with heart failure. N Engl J Med 2010;363(24):2301–9.

82. Koehler FF, Winkler SS, Schieber MM, et al. Tele-medical Interventional Monitoring in Heart Failure (TIM-HF), a randomized, controlled intervention trial investigating the impact of telemedicine on mortality in ambulatory patients with heart failure: study design. Eur J Heart Fail 2010;12(12): 1354–62.

83. Yancy CW, Jessup M, Bozkurt B, et al. 2013 ACCF/AHA Guideline for the Management of Heart Failure Association Task Force on Practice Guidelines. J Am Coll Cardiol 2013;62(16): e147–239.

84. Whellan DJ, Sarkar S, Koehler J, et al. Development of a method to risk stratify patients with heart failure for 30-day readmission using implantable device diagnostics. Am J Cardiol 2013;111(1): 79–84.

85. Ypenburg C, Bax JJ, van der Wall EE, et al. Intra-thoracic impedance monitoring to predict decompensated heart failure. Am J Cardiol 2007;99(4): 554–7.

86. Abraham WT, Adamson PB, Bourge RC, et al. Wireless pulmonary artery haemodynamic monitoring in chronic heart failure: a randomised controlled trial. Lancet 2011;377(9766):658–66.

87. Adamson PB, Abraham WT, Bourge RC, et al. Wireless pulmonary artery pressure monitoring guides management to reduce decompensation in heart failure with preserved ejection fraction. Circ Heart Fail 2014;7(6):935–44.

88. Gheorghiade MM, Pang PS, Ambrosy AP, et al. A comprehensive, longitudinal description of the in-hospital and post-discharge clinical, laboratory, and neurohormonal course of patients with heart failure who die or are re-hospitalized within 90 days: analysis from the EVEREST trial. Heart Fail Rev 2012;17(3):485–509.

89. Fonarow GC, Abraham WT, Albert NM, et al. Association between performance measures and clinical outcomes for patients hospitalized with heart failure. JAMA 2007;297(1):61–70.

90. Hernandez AF, Fonarow GC, Liang L, et al. The need for multiple measures of hospital quality: results from the Get with the Guidelines-Heart Failure Registry of the American Heart Association. Circulation 2011;124(6):712–9.

91. Felker GM, Lee KL, Bull DA, et al. Diuretic strategies in patients with acute decompensated heart failure. N Engl J Med 2011;364(9):797–805.

92. Cleland JG, McGowan J, Clark A, et al. The evidence for beta blockers in heart failure. BMJ 1999;318(7187):824–5.

93. Packer M, Coats AJ, Fowler MB, et al. Effect of carvedilol on survival in severe chronic heart failure. N Engl J Med 2001;344(22):1651–8.

94. Schrier RW, Gheorghiade M. Challenge of rehospitalizations for heart failure: potential of natriuretic doses of mineralocorticoid receptor antagonists. Am Heart J 2011;161(2):221–3.

95. The SOLVD Investigators. Effect of enalapril on mortality and the development of heart failure in asymptomatic patients with reduced left ventricular ejection fractions. N Engl J Med 1992;327(10): 685–91.

96. Zannad F, McMurray JJ, Krum H, et al. Eplerenone in patients with systolic heart failure and mild symptoms. N Engl J Med 2011;364:11–21.

97. Jong P, Demers C, McKelvie RS, et al. Angiotensin receptor blockers in heart failure: meta-analysis of

randomized controlled trials. J Am Coll Cardiol 2002;39(3):463–70.

98. Pitt B, Poole-Wilson PA, Segal R, et al. Effect of losartan compared with captopril on mortality in patients with symptomatic heart failure: randomised trial—the Losartan Heart Failure Survival Study ELITE II. Lancet 2000;355(9215):1582–7.

99. Gheorghiade M, Konstam MA, Burnett JC, et al. Short-term clinical effects of tolvaptan, an oral vasopressin antagonist, in patients hospitalized for heart failure: the EVEREST Clinical Status Trials. JAMA 2007;297(12):1332–43.

100. Schrier RW, Gross P, Gheorghiade M, et al. Tolvaptan, a selective oral vasopressin V2-receptor antagonist, for hyponatremia. N Engl J Med 2006; 355(20):2099–112.

101. Albert NM, Yancy CW, Liang L, et al. Use of aldosterone antagonists in heart failure. JAMA 2009; 302(15):1658–65.

102. Fonarow GC, Abraham WT, Albert NM, et al. Influence of a performance-improvement initiative on quality of care for patients hospitalized with heart failure results of the organized program to initiate lifesaving treatment in hospitalized patients with heart failure (OPTIMIZE-HF). Arch Intern Med 2007;167(14):1493–502.

103. Allen LA, Stevenson LW, Grady KL, et al. Decision making in advanced heart failure: a scientific statement from the American Heart Association. Circulation 2012;125(15):1928–52.

104. Casarett D, Pickard A, Bailey FA, et al. Do palliative consultations improve patient outcomes? J Am Geriatr Soc 2008;56(4):593–9.

105. Taylor AL, Ziesche S, Yancy C, et al. Combination of isosorbide dinitrate and hydralazine in blacks with heart failure. N Engl J Med 2004;351(20): 2049–57.

106. Morrison RS, Penrod JD, Cassel JB, et al. Cost savings associated with US hospital palliative care consultation programs. Arch Intern Med 2008;168(16):1783–90.

107. Norton SA, Hogan LA, Holloway RG, et al. Proactive palliative care in the medical intensive care unit: effects on length of stay for selected high-risk patients. Crit Care Med 2007;35(6):1530–5.

108. The Digitalis Investigation Group. The effect of digoxin on mortality and morbidity in patients with heart failure. N Engl J Med 1997;336(8):525–33.

109. Ahmed A, Rich MW, Fleg JL, et al. Effects of digoxin on morbidity and mortality in diastolic heart failure: the ancillary digitalis investigation group trial. Circulation 2006;114(5):397–403.

110. Bruce CR. A review of ethical considerations for ventricular assist device placement in older adults. Aging Dis 2013;4(2):100–12.

111. Bourge RC, Fleg JL, Fonarow GC, et al. Digoxin reduces 30-day all-cause hospital admission in older patients with chronic systolic heart failure. Am J Med 2013;126(8):701–8.

112. Ahmed A, Bourge RC, Fonarow GC, et al. Digoxin use and lower 30-day all-cause readmission for Medicare beneficiaries hospitalized for heart failure. Am J Med 2014;127(1):61–70.

113. Hashim T, Elbaz S, Patel K, et al. Digoxin and 30-day all-cause hospital admission in older patients with chronic diastolic heart failure. Am J Med 2014;127(2):132–9.

114. McMurray JJ, Packer M, Desai AS, et al. Angiotensin-neprilysin inhibition versus enalapril in heart failure. N Engl J Med 2014;371(11):993–1004.

115. Hernandez AF, Mi X, Hammill BG, et al. Associations between aldosterone antagonist therapy and risks of mortality and readmission among patients with heart failure and reduced ejection fraction. JAMA 2012;308(20):2097–107.

116. Califf RM, Vidaillet H, Goldman L. Advanced congestive heart failure: what do patients want? Am Heart J 1998;135(6 Pt 2 Su):S320–6.

117. Stanek EJ, Oates MB, McGhan WF, et al. Preferences for treatment outcomes in patients with heart failure: symptoms versus survival. J Card Fail 2000; 6:225–32.

118. Dev S, Clare RM, Felker GM, et al. Link between decisions regarding resuscitation and preferences for quality over length of life with heart failure. Eur J Heart Fail 2012;14(1):45–53.

119. Lewis EF, Johnson PA, Johnson W, et al. Preferences for quality of life or survival expressed by patients with heart failure. J Heart Lung Transplant 2001;20(9):1016–24.

120. MacIver J, Rao V, Delgado DH, et al. Choices: a study of preferences for end-of-life treatments in patients with advanced heart failure. J Heart Lung Transplant 2008;27(9):1002–7.

121. Yancy CW, Burnett JC, Fonarow GC, et al. Decompensated heart failure: is there a role for the outpatient use of nesiritide? Congest Heart Fail 2004; 10(5):230–6.

122. Felker GM, O'Connor CM, Braunwald E. Heart failure clinical research network investigators. Loop diuretics in acute decompensated heart failure: necessary? Evil? A necessary evil? Circ Heart Fail 2009;2(1):56–62.

123. Emerman CL, Demarco T, Costanzo MR, et al. Impact of intravenous diuretics on the outcomes of patients hospitalized with acute decompensated heart failure: insights from the ADHERE(R) Registry. J Card Fail 2004;10(4):S116.

124. Hebert KK, Dias AA, Franco EE, et al. Open access to an outpatient intravenous diuresis program in a systolic heart failure disease management program. Congest Heart Fail 2011;17(6):309–13.

125. Yancy CW, Krum H, Massie BM, et al. Safety and efficacy of outpatient nesiritide in patients with

advanced heart failure: results of the Second Follow-Up Serial Infusions of Nesiritide (FUSION II) trial. Circ Heart Fail 2008;1(1):9–16.

126. Ryder M, Murphy NF, McCaffrey D, et al. Outpatient intravenous diuretic therapy; potential for marked reduction in hospitalisations for acute decompensated heart failure. Eur J Heart Fail 2008;10(3): 267–72.

127. Lazkani M, Ota KS. The role of outpatient intravenous diuretic therapy in a transitional care program for patients with heart failure: a case series. J Clin Med Res 2012;4(6):434–8.

128. Zacharias H, Raw J, Nunn A, et al. Is there a role for subcutaneous furosemide in the community and hospice management of end-stage heart failure? Palliat Med 2011;25(6):658–63.

129. Banerjee P, Tanner G, Williams L. Intravenous diuretic day-care treatment for patients with heart failure. Clin Med 2012;12(2):133–6.

130. Costanzo MR, Mills RM, Wynne J. Characteristics of "Stage D" heart failure: insights from the Acute Decompensated Heart Failure National Registry Longitudinal Module (ADHERE LM). Am Heart J 2008;155(2):339–47.

131. Adler ED, Goldfinger JZ, Kalman J, et al. Palliative care in the treatment of advanced heart failure. Circulation 2009;120(25):2597–606.

132. Follath F, Yilmaz MB, Delgado JF, et al. Clinical presentation, management and outcomes in the Acute Heart Failure Global Survey of Standard Treatment (ALARM-HF). Intensive Care Med 2011; 37(4):619–26.

133. Guglin M, Kaufman M. Inotropes do not increase mortality in advanced heart failure. Int J Gen Med 2014;7:237–51.

134. Stevenson LW. Clinical use of inotropic therapy for heart failure: looking backward or forward? Part II: chronic inotropic therapy. Circulation 2003;108(4): 492–7.

135. Francis GS, Bartos JA, Adatya S. Inotropes. J Am Coll Cardiol 2014;63(20):2069–78.

136. Hershberger RE, Nauman D, Walker TL, et al. Care processes and clinical outcomes of continuous outpatient support with inotropes (COSI) in patients with refractory endstage heart failure. J Card Fail 2003;9(3):180–7.

137. Lyons MG, Carey L. Parenteral inotropic therapy in the home: an update for home care and hospice. Home Healthc Nurse 2013;31(4):190–206.

138. Cowley AJ, Skene AM. Treatment of severe heart failure: quantity or quality of life? A trial of enoximone. Enoximone Investigators. Br Heart J 1994; 72(3):226–30.

139. Packer M, Carver JR, Rodeheffer RJ, et al. Effect of oral milrinone on mortality in severe chronic heart failure. The PROMISE Study Research Group. N Engl J Med 1991;325(21):1468–75.

140. Packer M. The development of positive inotropic agents for chronic heart failure: how have we gone astray? J Am Coll Cardiol 1993;22(4 Suppl A):119A–26A.

141. Cohn JN, Goldstein SO, Greenberg BH, et al. A dose-dependent increase in mortality with vesnarinone among patients with severe heart failure. N Engl J Med 1998;339(25):1810–6.

142. Dies F, Krell M, Whitlow P. Intermittent, ambulatory dobutamine infusion in severe chronic cardiac failure. Br J Clin Pract 1986;45:37–40.

143. Oliva F, Latini R, Politi A, et al. Intermittent 6-month low-dose dobutamine infusion in severe heart failure: DICE multicenter trial. Am Heart J 1999; 138(2 Pt 1):247–53.

144. Miller LW, Merkle EJ, Herrmann V. Outpatient dobutamine for end-stage congestive heart failure. Crit Care Med 1990;18(1 Pt 2):S30–3.

145. Canver CC, Chanda J. Milrinone for long-term pharmacologic support of the status 1 heart transplant candidates. Ann Thorac Surg 2000;69(6):1823–6.

146. Brozena SC, Twomey C, Goldberg LR, et al. A prospective study of continuous intravenous milrinone therapy for status IB patients awaiting heart transplant at home. J Heart Lung Transplant 2004; 23(9):1082–6.

147. Upadya S, Lee FA, Saldarriaga C, et al. Home continuous positive inotropic infusion as a bridge to cardiac transplantation in patients with end-stage heart failure. J Heart Lung Transplant 2004; 23(4):466–72.

148. Sindone AP, Keogh AM, Macdonald PS, et al. Continuous home ambulatory intravenous inotropic drug therapy in severe heart failure: safety and cost efficacy. Am Heart J 1997;134(5 Pt 1):899–900.

149. Harjai KJ, Mehra MR, Ventura HO, et al. Home inotropic therapy in advanced heart failure: cost analysis and clinical outcomes. Chest 1997; 112(5):1298–303.

150. Hauptman PJ, Mikolajczak P, George A, et al. Chronic inotropic therapy in end-stage heart failure. Am Heart J 2006;152(6):1096.e1–8.

151. Gorodeski EZ, Chu EC, Reese JR, et al. Prognosis on chronic dobutamine or milrinone infusions for stage D heart failure. Circ Heart Fail 2009;2(4): 320–4.

152. Assad-Kottner C, Chen D, Jahanyar J, et al. The use of continuous milrinone therapy as bridge to transplant is safe in patients with short waiting times. J Card Fail 2008;14(10):839–43.

153. Meaux N. Home infusion of inotropic therapy for patients with advanced heart failure. Infusion 2012.

154. Rogers JG, Milano CA. Ramping up evidence-based ventricular assist device care. J Am Coll Cardiol 2012;1–2. http://dx.doi.org/10.1016/j.jacc.2012.08.978.

155. Demondion P, Fournel L, Niculescu M, et al. The challenge of home discharge with a total artificial heart: the La Pitie Salpetriere experience. European Journal of Cardio-Thoracic Surgery 2013; 44(5):843–8.

156. Kirklin JK, Naftel DC, Kormos RL, et al. Fifth INTERMACS annual report Risk factor analysis from more than 6,000 mechanical circulatory support patients. J Heart Lung Transplant 2013;32(2):141–56.

157. Kirklin JK, Naftel DC, Pagani FD, et al. Sixth INTERMACS annual report: a 10,000-patient database. J Heart Lung Transplant 2014;33(6):555–64.

158. Creaser JW, Rourke D, Vandenbogaart E, et al. Outcomes of biventricular mechanical support patients discharged to home to await heart transplantation. J Cardiovasc Nurs 2014. http://dx.doi.org/10.1097/JCN.0000000000000168.

159. Jaroszewski DE, Anderson EM, Pierce CN, et al. The SynCardia freedom driver: a portable driver for discharge home with the total artificial heart. J Heart Lung Transplant 2011;30(7):844–5.

160. El-Banayosy A, Kizner L, Arusoglu L, et al. Home discharge and out-of-hospital follow-up of total artificial heart patients supported by a portable driver system. ASAIO J 2014;60(2):148–53.

161. Dew MA, Kormos RL, Winowich S, et al. Quality of life outcomes in left ventricular assist system inpatients and outpatients. ASAIO J 1999;45(3):218–25.

162. Kwok T, Lee J, Woo J, et al. A randomized controlled trial of a community nurse-supported hospital discharge programme in older patients with chronic heart failure. J Clin Nurs 2008;17(1):109–17.

163. Göhler A, Januzzi JL, Worrell SS, et al. A systematic meta-analysis of the efficacy and heterogeneity of disease management programs in congestive heart failure. J Card Fail 2006;12(7):554–67.

164. Jovicic A, Holroyd-Leduc JM, Straus SE. Effects of self-management intervention on health outcomes of patients with heart failure: a systematic review of randomized controlled trials. BMC Cardiovasc Disord 2006;6:43.

165. Kim Y-J, Soeken KL. A meta-analysis of the effect of hospital-based case management on hospital length-of-stay and readmission. Nurs Res 2005; 54(4):255–64.

166. Phillips CO, Singa RM, Rubin HR, et al. Complexity of program and clinical outcomes of heart failure disease management incorporating specialist nurse-led heart failure clinics - a meta-regression analysis. Eur J Heart Fail 2005;7(3):9.

167. Roccaforte R, Demers C, Baldassarre F, et al. Effectiveness of comprehensive disease management programmes in improving clinical outcomes in heart failure patients. a meta-analysis. Eur J Heart Fail 2005;7(7):1133–44.

168. Taylor S, Bestall J, Cotter S, et al. Clinical service organisation for heart failure. Taylor SJ, ed. Cochrane Database Syst Rev. 2005;(2):CD002752–CD002752. http://dx.doi.org/10.1002/14651858.CD002752.pub2.

169. Gonseth J, Guallar-Castillón P, Banegas JR, et al. The effectiveness of disease management programmes in reducing hospital re-admission in older patients with heart failure: a systematic review and meta-analysis of published reports. Eur Heart J 2004;25(18):1570–95.

170. Gwadry-Sridhar FH, Flintoft V, Lee DS, et al. A systematic review and meta-analysis of studies comparing readmission rates and mortality rates in patients with heart failure. Arch Intern Med 2004;164(21):2315–20.

171. Phillips CO, Wright SM, Kern DE, et al. Comprehensive discharge planning with postdischarge support for older patients with congestive heart failure: a meta-analysis. JAMA 2004;291(11):1358–67.

172. McAlister FA, Lawson FM, Teo KK, et al. A systematic review of randomized trials of disease management programs in heart failure. Am J Med 2001;110(5):378–84.

Team-Based Care for Managing Cardiac Comorbidities in Heart Failure

Naveen Bellam, MD, MPH[a], Anita A. Kelkar, MD, MPH[b],
David J. Whellan, MD, MHS[a],*

KEYWORDS

- Heart failure • Cardiac comorbidities • Management • Affiliate providers • Multidisciplinary
- Team based

KEY POINTS

- Balancing HF and the multiple cardiac comorbidities remains difficult for any single provide.
- Collaboration between physicians, nurses, nurse practitioners, physician assistants, pharmacists, and other health care workers reduces the burden of care coordination and simultaneously improves delivery of care.
- Team-based approaches increase cost-effectiveness, reduce hospitalization rates, and equally important, give patients more resources and support, which research shows may ultimately improve compliance and outcomes.

INTRODUCTION

An anticipated 8 million adults will suffer from heart failure (HF) by 2030, an increase of 46% from 2010 numbers.[1] Although effective management involves appropriate medications[2–9] and other methods, including fluid and sodium restriction or even inotrope support,[4,5,10,11] simultaneously managing the patient's HF, cardiovascular comorbidities, and other needs in an aging population can be difficult for a single cardiologist. Affiliate providers and ancillary staff therefore have opportunities for larger roles in providing care in this patient population. Furthermore, initiatives in reducing readmission rates and appropriately using resources play an important role in health care delivery, thus creating impetus for re-evaluation of the current HF clinic treatment model. This article focuses on the management of cardiac comorbidities commonly seen in HF, with attention paid to the evidence supporting a multidisciplinary approach.

ATRIAL FIBRILLATION AND HEART FAILURE

Up to 50% of patients with severe HF develop atrial fibrillation (AF)[12]; conversely, AF is an independent risk factor for the development of HF.[13] AF increases the risk of thromboembolism, leading to many patients with HF receiving systemic anticoagulation. The required medications frequently cause lifestyle interferences including strict diet adherence and international normalized ratio (INR) monitoring to prevent bleeding or stroke. Adequate rate control, or in AF-induced HF, rhythm control, is another important issue requiring careful medication selection and titration. Although cardioversion remains an option as in all patients with atrial arrhythmias, antiarrhythmic medications should be considered, although amiodarone and dofetilide have the most widespread support in HF populations.[14] In patients with recurrent symptoms, the MAZE procedure or radiofrequency catheter ablation are additional options.

[a] Thomas Jefferson University, Department of Medicine, Philadelphia, PA, USA; [b] Emory University School of Medicine, Department of Medicine, Atlanta, GA, USA
* Corresponding author. 1015 Chestnut Street, Suite 317, Philadelphia, PA 19107.
E-mail address: david.whellan@jefferson.edu

Heart Failure Clin 11 (2015) 407–417
http://dx.doi.org/10.1016/j.hfc.2015.03.005

Specialty centers using a multidisciplinary approach have shown reductions in the incidence of AF-related hospitalizations and stroke.[15] Team-based care involves numerous stakeholders in patient care starting with the cardiologist, to nurse practitioners and pharmacists. For example, referral to electrophysiology for a study and/or ablation is now accepted care, because the 2014 American College of Cardiology (ACC) and American Heart Association (AHA) AF Guidelines have placed atrioventricular nodal ablation with permanent ventricular pacing as IIA recommendation for patients with HF for whom pharmacologic therapy is inadequate and rate control cannot be achieved.[16] These relationships not only improve outcomes in patients with AF, but also foster treatment strategies for patients whose AF cannot solely be managed by the general cardiologist.

Other health care workers, such as nurses, play key roles in multidisciplinary care. A study found that nurse-led care (consisting of guideline-based care supervised by cardiologists) compared with usual care of patients with AF significantly improved guideline adherence and the primary end point of composite cardiovascular hospitalization and hospitalized deaths at a 22-month follow-up.[17] Similar results were seen in the Standard Versus Atrial Fibrillation-Specific Management Strategy (SAFETY) study, a multicenter trial of 335 hospitalized patients with AF that randomized standard care (outpatient (primary care physician [PCP]) visit for follow-up) versus the SAFETY intervention (Holter monitor 7–14 days postdischarge, home cardiac nurse visits). The study showed prolonged days alive and days out of hospital in the SAFETY group compared with standard management.[18] Multiple studies have shown that nurse-coordinated care better organizes patient care, improves adherence to guideline recommendations, provides group education, and improves outcomes by providing close patient follow-up.[18,19]

Pharmacists also play unique roles in AF management by providing expertise in individualizing therapy based on patient-specific factors. The advances in novel anticoagulants allow pharmacists the ability to not only provide more customized medication selection, but also provide education on side effects, drug interactions, and make alternative strategies for anticoagulation or antiarrhythmics.[20] In those requiring warfarin, a retrospective cohort study of 179 patients using inpatient anticoagulation management services found a lower incidence of supratherapeutic INR and longer time within goal range in the pharmacist- versus physician-managed INR group.[21]

Ideally, a multidisciplinary approach to AF in patients with HF empowers and educates patients, while offering close follow-up, monitoring, and adequate and timely implementation and management of therapeutics. Such an approach not only improves AF-related morbidity and mortality, but also benefits patient-centered outcomes (**Fig. 1**).

ARRHYTHMIA MANAGEMENT AND HEART FAILURE

Conduction abnormalities and various cardiomyopathies can degenerate stable electrocardiographic rhythms into ventricular tachycardia or ventricular fibrillation, progressing to sudden cardiac death (SCD). With an incidence of approximately 3% annually,[13] options remain for prevention and improvement. These options include use of implantable cardioverter defibrillators (ICDs) in primary and secondary prevention of arrhythmias. When considering primary prevention of sudden death, ICDs have proven efficacy; the Multicenter Automatic Defibrillator Implantation Trial (MADIT II), a study of 1232 patients with left ventricular

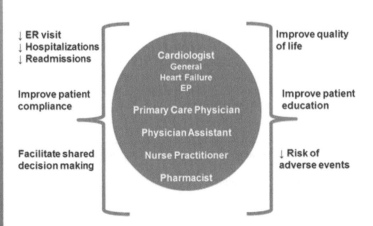

↓ ER visit
↓ Hospitalizations
↓ Readmissions

Improve patient compliance

Facilitate shared decision making

Cardiologist
General
Heart Failure
EP

Primary Care Physician

Physician Assistant

Nurse Practitioner

Pharmacist

Improve quality of life

Improve patient education

↓ Risk of adverse events

Fig. 1. Proposed atrial fibrillation multidisciplinary team and affected outcomes. EP, electrophysiology; ER, emergency room.

ejection fraction (LVEF) of less than 30% following myocardial infarction (MI), found a rate of SCD approximately 5.5% lower in patients with an ICD.[22] The Sudden Cardiac Death in Heart Failure Trial (SCD-HeFT) found overall mortality reduced with ICD use as well (29% vs 36%).[23]

Secondary prevention in patients with prior dangerous ventricular arrhythmias should also be recognized. Although many patients with ICDs eventually die from noncardiac causes, post hoc analyses have found ventricular tachycardia, ventricular fibrillation, and wide complex rhythms leading to electromechanical dissociation as a common cardiac cause of death.[24]

Catheter ablation of ventricular tachycardia also remains an option in three clinical situations: (1) as adjunct to ICD, (2) as an alternative to ICD (if not a candidate), and (3) as prophylactic adjunctive therapy along with ICD. Providers may also prescribe wearable cardioverter-defibrillators, with trained nurses completing fittings of the devices in patients requiring temporary protection, or during bridging periods; survival rates seem similar to that of ICD patients.[25] This option exists in the 40-day period following MI, because the DINAMIT trial showed survivors post-MI with low ejection fraction (EF) did not benefit from immediate ICD implantation.[26]

Affiliate providers help beyond device referral alone, because many procedures can cause fear and anxiety, and often require education and discussion. Nurses trained in providing telephone interventions following ICD placement found that patients had improved anxiety, knowledge, and reduced concerns regarding death.[27] Although the improvements did not translate into reductions in hospitalizations or provider visits, improved psychological profiles and better understanding of the disease process may improve patient satisfaction and trust, and create future gains when making recommendations in other areas of HF management.

CARDIAC RESYNCHRONIZATION THERAPY IN HEART FAILURE

Specific populations exhibiting HF symptoms despite optimal medical therapy benefit from cardiac resynchronization therapy, with pacing intended to improve ventricular electromechanical delay, also known as "dyssynchrony." Prolonged QRS duration along with dyssynchrony and impaired ventricular contraction are predictors of worsening HF, SCD, and increased mortality.[28] QRS durations greater than 120 milliseconds may exhibit dyssynchrony, but more commonly occurs when exceeding 150 milliseconds. Based

on existing data,[4] the ACC, AHA, and Heart Rhythm Society guidelines support device-based therapy with cardiac resynchronization therapy in patients in sinus rhythm with LVEF less than or equal to 35% as shown in **Table 1**.

Admissions regarding the management of ICDs are unfortunately not uncommon. The capability of these devices to continuously monitor heart rate, electrical disturbances, and abnormal rhythms can lead to scenarios ranging from audible notifications to electrical device discharge and defibrillation, in the case of ICDs. These events increase provider visits and hospitalizations, which may be unwanted or unnecessary at times. Among the multidisciplinary options available to care, one option evaluated remote monitoring in the Evolution of Management Strategies of Heart Failure with Implantable Defibrillators (EVOLVO) study. The trial randomized 200 patients with HF to remote monitoring versus standard patient visits, with a primary end point of urgent hospital or clinic visits. The remote monitoring arm used no audible patient alerts, and clinics checked the Medtronic (Minneapolis, MN) Carelink Web site daily for wirelessly transmitted events. The trial found a 35% reduction in unintended visits during the 16-month study period (**Fig. 2**) by using a wireless monitoring system.[29] Implementation of advanced monitoring systems for devices, blood pressure, and other aspects could reduce future visits and total health care use, and provide more timely evaluation of patient events.

MANAGING CORONARY ARTERY DISEASE AND HEART FAILURE

Although not considered a true cardiomyopathy by recent guidelines,[30,31] ischemic cardiomyopathy (ICM) is commonly defined as impaired left ventricular (LV) function in the setting of coronary artery disease (CAD). Although patients with non-ICM and nonobstructive disease have similar survival outcomes, data have identified worse outcomes when compared with ICM cohorts (**Fig. 3**), defined as patients with angiographically visualized stenosis within at least one major epicardial artery.[32] The 2013 AHA/ACC guidelines recommend coronary angiography for evaluation of the role of revascularization. One primary factor, however, differentiates true loss of myocardium and revascularization in ICM: viability. Recovery of the contractile function of myocardium remains an important factor in candidacy for revascularization, and guidelines support noninvasive evaluation of viability or myocardial ischemia in patients without angina.[4] Observational studies originally showed that revascularization in patients with

Table 1
2013 ACC/AHA/HRS guidelines for cardiac resynchronization therapy implantation

Class	Indication	Level of Evidence
Class 1	NYHA class II, III, or IV symptoms on GDMT, sinus rhythm, LBBB with a QRS duration ≥150 ms	Level of Evidence A for NYHA class III/IV Level of Evidence B in NYHA class II
Class 2A	NYHA class III/IV symptoms on GDMT with non-LBBB pattern and a QRS duration of ≥150 ms	Level of Evidence A
	NYHA class II, III, or IV symptoms on GDMT, with LBBB and a QRS duration 120–149 ms	Level of Evidence B
	On GDMT and undergoing placement of a new or replacement device with anticipated requirement for significant (>40%) ventricular pacing	Level of Evidence C
Class 2B	In patients with LVEF ≤30%, ischemic cause of heart failure, sinus rhythm and LBBB with a QRS duration ≥150 ms, and NYHA class I symptoms on GDMT	Level of Evidence C
	In patients with LVEF ≤35%, sinus rhythm and non-LBBB pattern with QRS duration 120–149 ms, and NYHA class III/IV symptoms on GDMT	Level of Evidence B
	In patients with LVEF ≤35%, sinus rhythm, a non-LBBB pattern with a QRS duration ≥150 ms, and NYHA class II symptoms on GDMT	Level of Evidence B
	In patients with LVEF ≤35%, sinus rhythm, a non-LBBB pattern with a QRS duration ≥150 ms, and NYHA class II symptoms on GDMT	Level of Evidence B
Class 3: No Benefit	Cardiac resynchronization therapy is not recommended for patients with NYHA class I or II symptoms and non-LBBB pattern with QRS duration <150 ms.	Level of Evidence B
	Cardiac resynchronization therapy is not indicated for patients whose comorbidities and/or frailty limit survival with good functional capacity to <1 y	Level of Evidence C

Abbreviations: GDMT, guideline-directed medical therapy; HRS, Heart Rhythm Society; LBBB, left bundle branch block; NYHA, New York Heart Association.

viability had improvements in LV function.[33] More recent randomized studies, however, suggest improvements in outcomes following revascularization may have less to do with LVEF, and more to do with improvements in care, medications, and preventing further worsening of existing disease.[34]

The benefits of coronary artery bypass grafting (CABG) in the setting of CAD have been studied for some time. Older studies related viable myocardium to improvements in LV function following surgery and improved survival,[35,36] along with reduced rates of future infarction.[37] More recently, the Surgical Treatment in Ischemic Heart Failure (STICH) trial evaluated the use of CABG in patients with CAD and HF.[38] The study randomized 1212 patients with an LVEF of less than 35% to medical therapy or medical therapy plus CABG. Although the findings included significant reductions in cardiovascular death or hospitalization (the secondary end point), the primary end point of overall deaths was nonsignificant (41% with medications vs 36% with CABG; P = .12, **Fig. 4**).

Criticisms, however, suggested that the lack of viability analysis affected outcomes. A subset analysis within STICH therefore answered the question of viability.[39] Although analysis initially found statistically significant differences in death rates, additional multivariate analysis showed no differences (P = .53; **Fig. 5**). The STICH trial subset also had smaller ventricular sizes at baseline, challenging the role of LV size.[40] Despite accounting for these factors, STICH still did not find a definite role for bypass surgery in those with HF.

Beyond surgery, minimal data exist for CABG versus percutaneous coronary intervention. Sedlis and colleagues[41] compared mortality outcomes between interventions in the Angina With Extremely Serious Operative Mortality Evaluation (AWESOME) trial, and found no difference

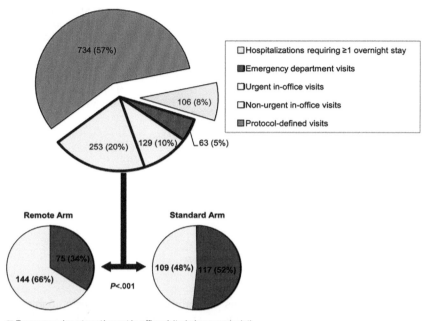

Fig. 2. EVOLVO study evaluating clinic or emergent visits using a remote (wireless clinic monitoring) versus standard device monitoring system. (*From* Landolina M, Perego GB, Lunati M, et al. Remote monitoring reduces healthcare use and improves quality of care in heart failure patients with implantable defibrillators: the Evolution of Management Strategies of Heart Failure Patients With Implantable Defibrillators (EVOLVO) study. Circulation 2012;125(24):2988; with permission.)

between groups in patients with an LVEF less than 35%. Importantly, the trial compared patients with angina and acute coronary syndrome; they did not evaluate improvements or outcomes related to HF itself. The advances in nonsurgical treatment options compared before STICH have likely attenuated some of the mortality benefits seen in earlier surgery trials. It is possible that younger patients, those without devices, or those unable to take all

recommended drug therapies may more likely benefit from surgery.

CAD in HF provides more prognostic information rather than therapeutic options. Studies have identified CAD as a predictor of higher mortality in patients with ICM, although no interventions have been shown to provide a benefit. Despite no clearly demonstrated benefits in revascularization, revascularization remains a class 2 indication

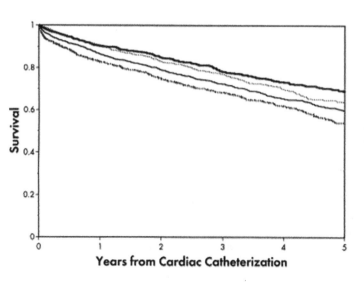

Fig. 3. Adjusted Kaplan-Meier survival estimates with nonischemic (*solid line*) and ischemic (*gray dashed line*) cardiomyopathies (*P*<.0001). (*From* Bart BA, Shaw LK, McCants CB Jr, et al. Clinical determinants of mortality in patients with angiographically diagnosed ischemic or nonischemic cardiomyopathy. J Am Coll Cardiol 1997;30(4):1006; with permission.)

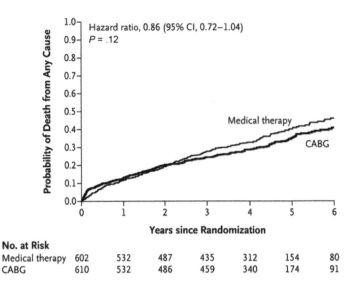

Fig. 4. STICH trial: Kaplan-Meier curves for the probability of death from any cause. CI, confidence interval. (*From* Velazquez EJ, Lee KL, Deja MA, et al. Coronary-artery bypass surgery in patients with left ventricular dysfunction. N Engl J Med 2011;364(17):1612; with permission.)

No. at Risk							
Medical therapy	602	532	487	435	312	154	80
CABG	610	532	486	459	340	174	91

in patients without angina. Current guidelines provide a class 1 recommendation for percutaneous or surgical revascularization in patients with HF only in the setting of angina, when suitable coronary anatomy exists, particularly left main stenosis or left main equivalent.[13]

Valvular heart disease in HF can range from asymptomatic disease to severe symptoms at

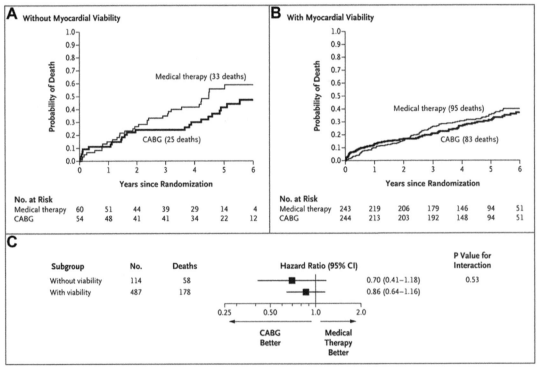

Fig. 5. STICH viability analysis: Kaplan-Meier analysis of the probability of death according to myocardial-viability status and treatment. (*A*) At 5 years, the rates of death for patients without myocardial viability were 41.5% in the group assigned to CABG and 55.8% in the group assigned to receive medical therapy. (*B*) Among patients with myocardial viability, the respective rates were 31.2% and 35.4%. (*C*) There was no significant interaction between viability status and treatment assignment with respect to mortality (*P* = .53). CI, confidence interval. (*From* Bonow RO, Maurer G, Lee KL, et al. Myocardial viability and survival in ischemic left ventricular dysfunction. N Engl J Med 2011;364(17):1623; with permission.)

rest. Research on repair or replacement of aortic and mitral valves has had mixed results, because patients with valvular surgery may have recurrence of HF symptoms as LV function declines and ventricular dilation ensues. Because valvular disease can cause and exacerbate HF, class II recommendations support valvular surgery.[4] Careful candidate selection is tantamount because reduced EF alone portends a poor prognosis for perioperative and postoperative mortality.

Decisions for surgery must also balance the risk of perioperative mortality. Assessment should consider use of the Gupta Peri-operative Cardiac Risk,[42] a calculator derived from a population of more than 400,000 patients. The predictive ability as measured by C statistic was 0.88 (88%), much higher than previous models, such as the Revised Cardiac Risk Index,[43] which has typically been the tool used by many physicians and anesthesiologists since the 1970s.

The nurse and nurse practitioner can also successfully fill in gaps following surgery and in transitions of care. One study found low mortality outcomes when transitioning from hospital to home in a nurse-led clinic of 1967 patients following acute coronary syndrome or bypass surgery when compared with usual clinic follow-up.[44] Hall and colleagues[45] found similar results; use of nurse practitioners reduced 30–day readmission and death rates with a "Follow Your Heart" home program. Patients receiving predischarge education, a telephone call within 24 hours, enrollment in a visiting nurse service, and a return clinic visit within 2 weeks had a 3.9% versus 11.5% readmission rate within 30 days ($P = .02$). This strategy may provide effective care, improve cost, and reduce complications following higher-risk interventions.

MANAGEMENT OF HYPERTENSION AND HEART FAILURE

Hypertension remains a common cause of HF in the United States[46]; approximately 5% of the more than 32,000 patients with hypertension developed HF in the ALLHAT trial.[47] This tasks the primary care physician or affiliate provider with recommending appropriate antihypertensive therapies that follow guidelines and provide mortality benefit wherever possible. Interestingly, however, higher baseline blood pressures have more favorable prognoses compared with normotensive patients. Metabolic, nutrition, and underlying inflammatory states are factors believed to predispose cardiac dysfunction and cause lower systemic pressures as part of the explanation for worse outcomes.[48] This paradox makes balancing hypertension management in HF more difficult than meets the eye.

Fortunately, most of the evidence-based treatments for heart failure with reduced left ventricular ejection fraction (HFrEF) also provide antihypertensive effects. β-Blocker therapy with the three medications of bisoprolol, carvedilol, and metoprolol succinate extended created long-term cardiovascular mortality relative reductions ranging from 31% to 44%,[7–9] with statistically significant findings for angiotensin-converting enzyme inhibitors and angiotensin receptor blockers.[49,50] Patients without compromised renal function or hyperkalemia, and EF of less than 35% with symptoms benefit from spironolactone as seen in the RALES study,[2] or with eplerenone for an EF less than 40% following MI, shown in the Epleronone Post-Acute Myocardial Infarction Heart Failure Efficacy and Survival Study (EPHUSES).[3] Mortality benefits ranged from 13% to 30% in these trials. Symptomatic African American patients with or without hypertension may benefit from hydralazine and nitrates based on data from the African American Heart Failure Trial (A-HeFT).[51] Diuretics commonly used to reduce fluid retention, edema, and symptoms may be chosen based on effectiveness, side effects, and resistance because little data exist to suggest one medication over another.

HYPERLIPIDEMIA IN HEART FAILURE

Hyperlipidemia remains a significant risk factor for HF, and aggressive statin treatment in patients with known CAD definitively reduces the risk of developing HF.[13] Even among patients without ischemic HF, statins improve mortality through pleotropic effects that not only lower cholesterol, but also impact cell death and decrease oxidative stress.[52] Paradoxically and despite the understanding of lipid management, baseline hypocholesterolemia represents a sign of increased mortality (**Fig. 6**) in patients with HF.[53] Current thoughts include mechanisms involving increased catabolism, inflammation, and immune dysregulation, similar to the dysfunction witnessed in septic populations.[54,55] At present, studies examining treatment of hyperlipidemia have had varied results in regards to statin therapy. One prospective cohort of 551 patients with ischemic and nonischemic systolic HF (EF <40%) investigating the impact of statin therapy found that treatment remained an independent predictor of improved survival (hazard ratio, 0.41; 95% confidence interval, 0.18–0.94) even after adjusting for risk factors, such as age and CAD.[56] Another meta-analysis found similar improved survival rates in patients with HF and preserved EF.[57] In contrast, the CORONA trial did not

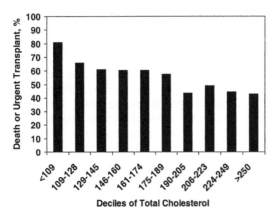

Fig. 6. Five-year rates of death or urgent heart transplantation by deciles of total cholesterol in heart failure. (*From* Horwich TB, Fonarow GC, Hamilton MA, et al. Low serum total cholesterol is associated with marked increase in mortality in advanced heart failure. J Card Fail 2002;8(4):222; with permission.)

find mortality improvements in patients with symptomatic systolic HF (hazard ratio, 0.92; 95% confidence interval, 0.83–1.02; P = .12).[58] Although randomized trials of routine statin use have not shown a definite mortality benefit in HF populations with hyperlipidemia,[58,59] aggressive control is still status quo for improving clinical outcomes. Further research must continue in this area.

MISCELLANEOUS TEAM-BASED AND MULTIDISCIPLINARY APPROACHES TO CARDIAC COMORBIDITIES IN HEART FAILURE

The team-based approach to managing patients with HF remains underused despite ACC/AHA recommendations.[60] The combination of an aging population with multiple comorbidities, pressures within the clinic, and initiatives to reduce HF readmissions have placed immense stresses on the physician provider. Ultimately, an affiliate provider-staffed clinic can improve options and time management for cardiology practices without placing excess pressure on a single physician.

The multimodal benefits of affiliate providers in the nonacademic outpatient setting were proved in the Improve the Use of Evidence-Based Heart Failure Therapies in the Outpatient Setting (IMPROVE-HF) Registry, which prospectively enrolled 167 cardiology practices involving 15,381 patients with chronic HF and an LVEF less than 35%, and examined adherence to guideline-driven medication recommendations, device use, and HF education. The results showed that clinics employing physician groups with affiliate providers performed equally well in adhering to guidelines versus physicians alone.[61] Additionally, authors Albert and colleagues[61] identified a

trend toward significance in providing HF education in the affiliate provider cohort (P = .08). They suggested that better patient education may improve decision making and provider-patient trust, and could affect management during hospitalization or better navigate complex discussions related to end-of-life care.

Nurse-led clinics have had great success in medication titration, because maximum β-blocker dosing was shorter in nurse-led groups versus usual clinic care.[62] Usage of nurse-managed clinics also showed cost effectiveness[63] and improvements in hospitalization rates.[64] Opportunities for home visits or travel to rural settings exist, and telephone-based disease management is also an option, but data seem mixed at present.[65] These approaches may need further study.

UNDERSTANDING THE ROLE OF CLINICAL TRIALS IN MANAGING CARDIAC MORBIDITIES IN HEART FAILURE

The enforcement of recommendations in research trials and compliance with existing regimens when managing cardiovascular comorbidities can also improve outcomes. This was demonstrated by the HF-ACTION trial, which randomized 2331 patients with HF to a formal supervised exercise program thrice-weekly or to usual care and evaluated the safety and efficacy of structured exercise.[66] Patients assigned to the usual care group received educational, HF, diet, and exercise (30 minutes most days) recommendations per guidelines. When adjusting for predictive risk factors, the study had a modest effect on overall cardiovascular or mortality outcomes. Equally interesting, however, a survey showed 55% of patients in the usual care group were unsatisfied with their randomization, leading to some crossover. In addition, HF-ACTION had a guideline-directed compliance rate of 95% for patients without contraindications. Such numbers are essentially unheard of in settings lacking close follow-up and oversight. Research settings provide added safety monitoring systems and oversight, enabling the clinician to reach medication or intervention goals while reducing adverse risk. Without adequate support systems, many patients have difficulty attaining the efficacy end points seen in many evidenced-based trials.

SUMMARY

The need for HF management is predicted to increase as the HF population ages. Balancing HF and the multiple cardiac comorbidities remains difficult for any single provider, but becomes easier with the involvement of a team. Collaboration between physicians, nurses, nurse practitioners, physician assistants, pharmacists, and other health care workers reduces the burden of care coordination and simultaneously improves delivery of care. Team-based approaches increase cost-effectiveness, reduce hospitalization rates, and equally important, give patients more resources and support, which research shows may ultimately improve compliance and outcomes.

REFERENCES

1. Heidenreich PA, Albert NM, Allen LA, et al. Forecasting the impact of heart failure in the United States: a policy statement from the American Heart Association. Circ Heart Fail 2013;6(3):606–19.
2. Pitt B, Zannad F, Remme WJ, et al. The effect of spironolactone on morbidity and mortality in patients with severe heart failure. Randomized aldactone evaluation study investigators. N Engl J Med 1999; 341(10):709–17.
3. Pitt B, Remme W, Zannad F, et al. Eplerenone, a selective aldosterone blocker, in patients with left ventricular dysfunction after myocardial infarction. N Engl J Med 2003;348(14):1309–21.
4. Yancy CW, Jessup M, Bozkurt B, et al. 2013 ACCF/AHA guideline for the management of heart failure: executive summary: a report of the American College of Cardiology Foundation/American Heart Association Task Force on practice guidelines. Circulation 2013;128(16):1810–52.
5. Heart Failure Society of America, Lindenfeld J, Albert NM, et al. HFSA 2010 comprehensive heart failure practice guideline. J Card Fail 2010;16(6): e1–194.
6. The Cardiac Insufficiency Bisoprolol Study II (CIBIS-II): a randomised trial. Lancet 1999;353(9146):9–13.
7. Dargie HJ. Effect of carvedilol on outcome after myocardial infarction in patients with left-ventricular dysfunction: the CAPRICORN randomised trial. Lancet 2001;357(9266):1385–90.
8. A randomized trial of beta-blockade in heart failure. The Cardiac Insufficiency Bisoprolol Study (CIBIS). CIBIS Investigators and Committees. Circulation 1994;90(4):1765–73.
9. Effect of metoprolol CR/XL in chronic heart failure: Metoprolol CR/XL Randomised Intervention Trial in Congestive Heart Failure (MERIT-HF). Lancet 1999; 353:2001–7.
10. Travers B, O'Loughlin C, Murphy NF, et al. Fluid restriction in the management of decompensated heart failure: no impact on time to clinical stability. J Card Fail 2007;13(2):128–32.
11. Aliti GB, Rabelo ER, Clausell N, et al. Aggressive fluid and sodium restriction in acute decompensated heart failure: a randomized clinical trial. JAMA Intern Med 2013;173(12):1058–64.
12. Maisel WH, Stevenson LW. Atrial fibrillation in heart failure: epidemiology, pathophysiology, and rationale for therapy. Am J Cardiol 2003;91(6 Suppl 1):2–8.
13. Yancy CW, Jessup M, Bozkurt B, et al. 2013 ACCF/AHA guideline for the management of heart failure: a report of the American College of Cardiology Foundation/American Heart Association Task Force on Practice Guidelines. J Am Coll Cardiol 2013; 62(16):e147–239.
14. January CT, Wann LS, Alpert JS, et al. 2014 AHA/ACC/HRS Guideline for the management of patients with atrial fibrillation: a report of the American College of Cardiology/American Heart Association Task Force on Practice Guidelines and the Heart Rhythm Society. Circulation 2014;130:2071–104.
15. Tran HN, Tafreshi J, Hernandez EA, et al. A multidisciplinary atrial fibrillation clinic. Curr Cardiol Rev 2013;9(1):55–62.
16. January CT, Wann LS, Alpert JS, et al. 2014 AHA/ACC/HRS Guideline for the management of patients with atrial fibrillation: executive summary: a report of the American College of Cardiology/American Heart Association Task Force on Practice Guidelines and the Heart Rhythm Society. J Am Coll Cardiol 2014; 64(21):2246–80.
17. Hendriks JM, de Wit R, Crijns HJ, et al. Nurse-led care vs. usual care for patients with atrial fibrillation: results of a randomized trial of integrated chronic care vs. routine clinical care in ambulatory patients with atrial fibrillation. Eur Heart J 2012;33(21):2692–9.
18. Stewart S, Ball J, Horowitz J. Standard versus atrial fibrillation-specific management strategy (SAFETY) to reduce recurrent admission and prolong survival: pragmatic, multicentre, randomised controlled trial. Lancet 2014;385 [pii:S0140-6736(14)61992-9].
19. Berti D, Hendriks JM, Brandes A, et al. A proposal for interdisciplinary, nurse-coordinated atrial fibrillation expert programmes as a way to structure daily practice. Eur Heart J 2013;34:2725–30.
20. Practice spotlight: pharmacists in a multidisciplinary atrial fibrillation clinic. Can J Hosp Pharm 2011; 64(5):370–1.
21. Chilipko AA, Norwood DK. Evaluating warfarin management by pharmacists in a community teaching hospital. Consult Pharm 2014;29(2):95–103.
22. Moss AJ, Zareba W, Hall WJ, et al. Prophylactic implantation of a defibrillator in patients with myocardial infarction and reduced ejection fraction. N Engl J Med 2002;346(12):877–83.
23. Bardy GH, Lee KL, Mark DB, et al. Amiodarone or an implantable cardioverter-defibrillator for congestive heart failure. N Engl J Med 2005;352(3):225–37.
24. Grubman EM, Pavri BB, Shipman T, et al. Cardiac death and stored electrograms in patients with

third-generation implantable cardioverter-defibrillators. J Am Coll Cardiol 1998;32(4):1056–62.

25. Chung MK, Szymkiewicz SJ, Shao M, et al. Aggregate national experience with the wearable cardioverter-defibrillator: event rates, compliance, and survival. J Am Coll Cardiol 2010;56(3):194–203.

26. Hohnloser SH, Kuck KH, Dorian P, et al. Prophylactic use of an implantable cardioverter-defibrillator after acute myocardial infarction. N Engl J Med 2004; 351(24):2481–8.

27. Dougherty CM, Thompson EA, Lewis FM. Long-term outcomes of a telephone intervention after an ICD. Pacing Clin Electrophysiol 2005;28(11):1157–67.

28. Naccarelli GV, Luck JC, Wolbrette DL, et al. Pacing therapy for congestive heart failure: is it ready for prime time? Curr Opin Cardiol 1999;14(1):1–3.

29. Landolina M, Perego GB, Lunati M, et al. Remote monitoring reduces healthcare use and improves quality of care in heart failure patients with implantable defibrillators: the evolution of management strategies of heart failure patients with implantable defibrillators (EVOLVO) study. Circulation 2012; 125(24):2985–92.

30. Maron BJ, Towbin JA, Thiene G, et al. Contemporary definitions and classification of the cardiomyopathies: an American Heart Association Scientific Statement from the Council on Clinical Cardiology, Heart Failure and Transplantation Committee; Quality of Care and Outcomes Research and Functional Genomics and Translational Biology Interdisciplinary Working Groups; and Council on Epidemiology and Prevention. Circulation 2006;113:1807–16.

31. Elliott P, Andersson B, Arbustini E, et al. Classification of the cardiomyopathies: a position statement from the European Society Of Cardiology Working Group on Myocardial and Pericardial Diseases. Eur Heart J 2008;29(2):270–6.

32. Bart BA, Shaw LK, McCants CB Jr, et al. Clinical determinants of mortality in patients with angiographically diagnosed ischemic or nonischemic cardiomyopathy. J Am Coll Cardiol 1997;30(4):1002–8.

33. Allman KC, Shaw LJ, Hachamovitch R, et al. Myocardial viability testing and impact of revascularization on prognosis in patients with coronary artery disease and left ventricular dysfunction: a meta-analysis. J Am Coll Cardiol 2002;39(7):1151–8.

34. Holper EM, Blair J, Selzer F, et al. The impact of ejection fraction on outcomes after percutaneous coronary intervention in patients with congestive heart failure: an analysis of the National Heart, Lung, and Blood Institute Percutaneous Transluminal Coronary Angioplasty Registry and Dynamic Registry. Am Heart J 2006;151(1):69–75.

35. O'Connor CM, Velazquez EJ, Gardner LH, et al. Comparison of coronary artery bypass grafting versus medical therapy on long-term outcome in patients with ischemic cardiomyopathy (a 25-year experience from the Duke Cardiovascular Disease Databank). Am J Cardiol 2002;90(2):101–7.

36. Ragosta M, Beller GA, Watson DD, et al. Quantitative planar rest-redistribution 201Tl imaging in detection of myocardial viability and prediction of improvement in left ventricular function after coronary bypass surgery in patients with severely depressed left ventricular function. Circulation 1993;87(5):1630–41.

37. Samady H, Elefteriades JA, Abbott BG, et al. Failure to improve left ventricular function after coronary revascularization for ischemic cardiomyopathy is not associated with worse outcome. Circulation 1999;100(12):1298–304.

38. Velazquez EJ, Lee KL, Deja MA, et al. Coronary-artery bypass surgery in patients with left ventricular dysfunction. N Engl J Med 2011;364(17):1607–16.

39. Bonow RO, Maurer G, Lee KL, et al. Myocardial viability and survival in ischemic left ventricular dysfunction. N Engl J Med 2011;364(17):1617–25.

40. Schinkel AF, Poldermans D, Rizzello V, et al. Why do patients with ischemic cardiomyopathy and a substantial amount of viable myocardium not always recover in function after revascularization? J Thorac Cardiovasc Surg 2004;127(2):385–90.

41. Sedlis SP, Ramanathan KB, Morrison DA, et al. Outcome of percutaneous coronary intervention versus coronary bypass grafting for patients with low left ventricular ejection fractions, unstable angina pectoris, and risk factors for adverse outcomes with bypass (the AWESOME Randomized Trial and Registry). Am J Cardiol 2004;94(1):118–20.

42. Gupta PK, Gupta H, Sundaram A, et al. Development and validation of a risk calculator for prediction of cardiac risk after surgery. Circulation 2011;124(4): 381–7.

43. Goldman L, Caldera DL, Nussbaum SR, et al. Multifactorial index of cardiac risk in noncardiac surgical procedures. N Engl J Med 1977;297(16):845–50.

44. Wit MA, Bos-Schaap AJ, Hautvast RW, et al. Nursing role to improve care to infarct patients and patients undergoing heart surgery: 10 years' experience. Neth Heart J 2012;20(1):5–11.

45. Hall MH, Esposito RA, Pekmezaris R, et al. Cardiac surgery nurse practitioner home visits prevent coronary artery bypass graft readmissions. Ann Thorac Surg 2014;97(5):1488–93 [discussion: 1493–5].

46. Levy D, Larson MG, Vasan RS, et al. The progression from hypertension to congestive heart failure. JAMA 1996;275(20):1557–62.

47. Piller LB, Baraniuk S, Simpson LM, et al. Long-term follow-up of participants with heart failure in the antihypertensive and lipid-lowering treatment to prevent heart attack trial (ALLHAT). Circulation 2011;124: 1811–8.

48. Kalantar-Zadeh K, Block G, Horwich T, et al. Reverse epidemiology of conventional cardiovascular risk

factors in patients with chronic heart failure. J Am Coll Cardiol 2004;43(8):1439–44.

49. Granger CB, McMurray JJ, Yusuf S, et al. Effects of candesartan in patients with chronic heart failure and reduced left-ventricular systolic function intolerant to angiotensin-converting-enzyme inhibitors: the CHARM-Alternative trial. Lancet 2003; 362(9386):772–6.

50. Effect of enalapril on survival in patients with reduced left ventricular ejection fractions and congestive heart failure. The SOLVD Investigators. N Engl J Med 1991;325(5):293–302.

51. Taylor AL, Ziesche S, Yancy C, et al. Combination of isosorbide dinitrate and hydralazine in blacks with heart failure. N Engl J Med 2004;351:2049–57.

52. Swenne CA. Beyond lipid lowering: pleiotropic effects of statins in heart failure. Neth Heart J 2013;21(9):406–7.

53. Horwich TB, Hamilton MA, Maclellan WR, et al. Low serum total cholesterol is associated with marked increase in mortality in advanced heart failure. J Card Fail 2002;8(4):216–24.

54. Rauchhaus M, Koloczek V, Volk H, et al. Inflammatory cytokines and the possible immunological role for lipoproteins in chronic heart failure. Int J Cardiol 2000;76(2–3):125–33.

55. von Haehling S, Schefold JC, Springer J, et al. The cholesterol paradox revisited: heart failure, systemic inflammation, and beyond. Heart Fail Clin 2008;4(2): 141–51.

56. Horwich TB, MacLellan WR, Fonarow GC. Statin therapy is associated with improved survival in ischemic and non-ischemic heart failure. J Am Coll Cardiol 2004;43(4):642–8.

57. Liu G, Zheng XX, Xu YL, et al. Meta-analysis of the effect of statins on mortality in patients with preserved ejection fraction. Am J Cardiol 2014;113(7): 1198–204.

58. Kjekshus J, Apetrei E, Barrios V, et al. Rosuvastatin in older patients with systolic heart failure. N Engl J Med 2007;357(22):2248–61.

59. Gissi HF, Tavazzi L, Maggioni AP, et al. Effect of rosuvastatin in patients with chronic heart failure (the GISSI-HF trial): a randomised, double-blind, placebo-controlled trial. Lancet 2008;372(9645): 1231–9.

60. Jessup M, Abraham WT, Casey DE, et al. 2009 focused update: ACCF/AHA Guidelines for the Diagnosis and Management of Heart Failure in Adults: a report of the American College of Cardiology Foundation/American Heart Association Task Force on Practice Guidelines: developed in collaboration with the International Society for Heart and Lung Transplantation. Circulation 2009;119(14): 1977–2016.

61. Albert NM, Fonarow GC, Yancy CW, et al. Outpatient cardiology practices with advanced practice nurses and physician assistants provide similar delivery of recommended therapies (findings from IMPROVE HF). Am J Cardiol 2010;105(12):1773–9.

62. Driscoll A, Srivastava P, Toia D, et al. A nurse-led up-titration clinic improves chronic heart failure optimization of beta-adrenergic receptor blocking therapy: a randomized controlled trial. BMC Res Notes 2014; 7(1):668.

63. Henrick A. Cost-effective outpatient management of persons with heart failure. Prog Cardiovasc Nurs 2001;16(2):50–6.

64. Branch RD Jr. A CHF clinic. How aggressive outpatient care can offset hospitalization. JAAPA 1999; 12(10):24–6, 29, 32 passim.

65. Dunagan WC, Littenberg B, Ewald GA, et al. Randomized trial of a nurse-administered, telephone-based disease management program for patients with heart failure. J Card Fail 2005;11(5): 358–65.

66. O'Connor CM, Whellan DJ, Lee KL, et al. Efficacy and safety of exercise training in patients with chronic heart failure: HF-ACTION randomized controlled trial. JAMA 2009;301(14):1439–50.

Team-Based Care for Managing Noncardiac Conditions in Patients with Heart Failure

Justin M. Vader, MD, Michael W. Rich, MD*

KEYWORDS

- Heart failure • Noncardiac comorbidity • Team-based care • Multimorbidity • Geriatric

KEY POINTS

- Noncardiac comorbidity is present in most patients with heart failure (HF), and more than 50% have 4 or greater noncardiac conditions.
- Noncardiac comorbidities are associated with adverse outcomes in HF, particularly chronic kidney disease, chronic obstructive pulmonary disease, dementia, malignancy, and depression.
- Team-based care strategies improve process measures and outcomes in noncardiac conditions, but the efficacy of these interventions in the setting of coexisting HF requires further study.

INTRODUCTION

Heart failure (HF) affects 5.1 million Americans, with a mortality rate approaching 50% at 5 years, a major burden of morbidity and hospitalization,[1] and total costs estimated at $32 billion per year.[2] Although there are no proven therapies for reducing morbidity and mortality in HF with preserved ejection fraction (HFpEF), patients with HF with reduced ejection fraction (HFrEF) treated with guideline-recommended drug and device therapies experience greatly improved quality of life and reduced mortality and hospitalization.[3] Such a prevalent, mortal, morbid, expensive but modifiable disease state with care administered across multiple environments is a natural fit for highly integrated team-based care strategies. Moreover, HF rarely stands alone. Cardiovascular comorbidities contribute to the development of and progression of HF; guideline recommendations exist for these conditions, including coronary artery disease, atrial and ventricular arrhythmias, valvular heart disease, peripheral vascular

disease, and cerebrovascular disease. However, guidance on the comanagement of noncardiac comorbidities, equally if not more prevalent than cardiac comorbidities, is largely absent from practice guidelines; key knowledge gaps exist in the interplay of noncardiac comorbidity and HF.

NONCARDIAC COMORBIDITY IN PATIENTS WITH HEART FAILURE
Prevalence

HF prevalence increases with age; thus, Medicare represents the major payer for HF in the United States. The 14% of Medicare beneficiaries with HF account for 43% of Medicare Part A and Part B expenditures.[4] HF in the absence of noncardiovascular comorbidity among Medicare beneficiaries is *very rare*, occurring in only 4% of patients with HF. More than 50% of Medicare patients with HF have 4 or more noncardiovascular comorbidities and more than 25% have 6 or more.[5] The most prevalent noncardiac comorbidities include hypertension, hyperlipidemia, anemia,

Disclosures: Research support NHLBI Heart Failure Network (J.M. Vader); none (M.W. Rich).
Division of Cardiology, Washington University School of Medicine, 660 South Euclid Avenue, Campus Box 8086, St Louis, MO 63110, USA
* Corresponding author.
E-mail address: mrich@wustl.edu

Heart Failure Clin 11 (2015) 419–429
http://dx.doi.org/10.1016/j.hfc.2015.03.006
1551-7136/15/$ – see front matter © 2015 Elsevier Inc. All rights reserved.

heartfailure.theclinics.com

diabetes, arthritis, chronic kidney disease (CKD), chronic respiratory conditions, depression, and dementia (**Table 1**). Furthermore, data from the National Health and Nutrition Examination Survey (NHANES) indicate that the burden of comorbidity is growing, with the prevalence of 5 or more comorbidities in HF increasing from 42% in 1988 to 1994 to 58% in 2003 to 2008 (**Fig. 1**) and the mean number of prescriptions increasing from 4.1 to 6.4 per patient.[6] Noncardiac comorbidities particularly increase as a function of age, though in the oldest old the greater prevalence of conditions such as dementia is offset by a lower prevalence of diabetes.[7] In European patients with HF, comorbidities may be less prevalent (or less frequently diagnosed); but 43% of patients in a large European HF cohort had 2 or more comorbidities.[8]

Outcomes

Braunstein and colleagues[5] analyzed the risk ratio of various noncardiovascular comorbidities in relation to ambulatory-care sensitive HF hospitalizations (ie, potentially preventable through optimal primary care delivery) in Medicare patients with HF and found that the highest risks for such hospitalizations were in those with renal failure, hypertension, obstructive lung disease, lower

respiratory illness, and diabetes. Meanwhile, risk of death was greatest for lower respiratory illness, renal failure, dementia, cerebrovascular disease, and depression. The risks posed by specific comorbidities for hospitalization and overall mortality were not necessarily concordant (eg, dementia was associated with greater mortality but less hospitalization). In a separate multivariate analysis of mortality among Medicare/Medicaid beneficiaries with HF, the conditions contributing the highest hazard for death were lung and colorectal cancer, CKD, dementia, and chronic obstructive pulmonary disease (COPD), whereas the effect of diabetes was modest. In comparing hospitalized versus nonhospitalized patients with HF, noncardiovascular comorbidity contributed a relatively greater hazard of death among nonhospitalized patients with HF, suggesting that in those with less advanced HF, attention to noncardiac comorbidity might be relatively more important (**Table 2**).[9]

Noncardiac Comorbidity in Heart Failure with Preserved Versus Reduced Ejection Fraction

Noncardiac comorbidities in HFpEF and HFrEF differ in terms of prevalence and influence on outcomes.[10] A systematic review of studies comparing HFpEF with HFrEF showed higher prevalence of certain noncardiovascular comorbidities in HFpEF, particularly hypertension, renal impairment, chronic lung diseases, anemia, cancer, liver disease, peptic ulcer disease, and hypothyroidism.[11] Overall, all-cause mortality in patients with HFpEF is minimally if at all better than in patients with HFrEF.[12–14] Although some data suggest noncardiovascular causes of death are relatively more common in HFpEF compared with HFrEF,[15] reported rates of noncardiovascular death in HFpEF vary widely, ranging from 20% to 49%, perhaps because of the variability in cause-specific death reporting or definition of HFpEF.[11] In a largely male cohort, HFpEF compared with HFrEF was associated with more noncardiovascular comorbidities, particularly diabetes, anemia, COPD, obesity, cancer, and psychiatric disorders. In this study, HFpEF subjects had lower overall mortality and HF hospitalization but higher non-HF hospitalization. The contribution of various comorbidities to the hazard of death was similar between HFrEF and HFpEF, except for COPD, which was associated with a greater hazard for death in HFpEF.[16]

Table 1 Prevalence of selected noncardiac comorbidities in HF	
	Age <65 y
COPD	33%
Arthritis	35%
Depression	36%
CKD	45%
Diabetes	59%
Hypertension	81%
	Age ≥65 y
Dementia	28%
COPD	30%
CKD	42%
Arthritis	44%
Diabetes	46%
Hypertension	84%

Medicare data, 2011.

Abbreviation: COPD, chronic obstructive pulmonary disease.

From Yancy CW, Jessup M, Bozkurt B, et al. 2013 ACCF/AHA guideline for the management of heart failure: a report of the American College of Cardiology Foundation/American Heart Association Task Force on Practice Guidelines. Circulation 2013;128(16):e294; with permission.

THE ROLE OF TEAM-BASED CARE IN NONCARDIAC COMORBID CONDITIONS

As described elsewhere in this edition of *Heart Failure Clinics*, and as adopted by the Institute of

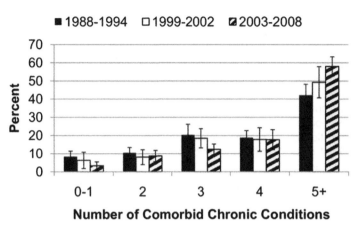

Fig. 1. Trends in number of comorbid conditions in patients with HF from NHANES. (*From* Wong CY, Chaudhry SI, Desai MM, et al. Trends in comorbidity, disability, and polypharmacy in heart failure. Am J Med 2011;124(2):140; with permission.)

Medicine in their *Core Principles & Values of Effective Team-Based Health Care*,[17] team-based health care is the provision of health services to individuals, families, and/or their communities by at least 2 health providers who work collaboratively with patients and their caregivers, to the extent preferred by each patient, to accomplish shared goals within and across settings to achieve coordinated high-quality care.[18] The role of team-based care in managing noncardiac comorbidities prevalent in the HF population is reviewed later.

Hypertension

Hypertension is well suited to team-based intervention. Contemporary hypertension guidelines[19] endorse the "2013 (American College of Cardiology/American Heart Association) ACC/AHA Guideline on Lifestyle Management to Reduce Cardiovascular Risk,"[20] creating an opportunity for dieticians, trainers, physical therapists, and exercise physiologists to contribute to favorable outcomes. Pharmacotherapy is goal directed, requiring dose titration and attention to pharmacodynamics and pharmacokinetics as well as intraindividual and interindividual variability of drug effects, creating a need for office and home-based nursing, pharmacist consultation, patient education, patient self-monitoring, and potentially remote monitoring strategies. Quality-improvement strategies that include adoption of multidisciplinary care teams result in the greatest improvements in blood pressure (BP).[21] In clinical trials using team-based care, greater likelihood of controlled BP was seen in studies involving nurses, clinic-based pharmacists, and community pharmacists (in order of increasing benefit).[22] Strategies using pharmacist recommendations to physicians, counseling on lifestyle modification, pharmacist-led interventions, and algorithm use were associated with the greatest benefits. Finally, regular review of patient charts with an associated stepped-care approach to pharmacotherapy is effective for lowering BP; interventions using nurse or pharmacist-based care seem to be particularly effective.[23]

Although these trials in hypertension were in the setting of the prevention of heart disease as

Table 2
Effect of burden of comorbidity on mortality among beneficiaries with HF

	Adjusted Hazard Ratio (95% CI)		Interaction Between Hospitalization Status & Comorbidity Burden
Burden of Comorbidity	Hospitalized Beneficiaries	Nonhospitalized Beneficiaries	P Value
Low (≤2 conditions)	1.0 (Reference)	1.0 (Reference)	—
Medium (3–4 conditions)	1.22 (1.13, 1.31)	1.49 (1.39,1.59)	.0003
High (≥5 conditions)	1.57 (1.44, 1.68)	2.35 (2.17, 2.54)	<.0001

Adjusted for age, sex, and race.
Abbreviation: CI, confidence interval.
From Ahluwalia SC, Gross CP, Chaudhry SI, et al. Impact of comorbidity on mortality among older persons with advanced heart failure. J Gen Intern Med 2012;27(5):516; with permission.

opposed to the therapy for HF, the principles of organized or protocol-driven patient review with stepped pharmacotherapy using the assistance of nurses and pharmacists has a direct application to the titration of HF pharmacotherapy. Pharmacist-led titration has been shown to increase the percentage of patients receiving optimal HF drug dosing,[24] and nurse-led phone-based intervention may increase both the proportion of patients achieving the trial-defined optimal dose and may improve left ventricular ejection fraction and reduce the need for device therapy in HF.[25]

Diabetes

Diabetes is present in more than one-third of Medicare recipients with HF.[5] The literature supports a role for poor diabetes control in the development of worsening HF in both patients with type I diabetes and patients with type II diabetes.[26–28] Although diabetes is a risk factor for HF hospitalization, its contribution to overall mortality is modest compared with other comorbidities.[5,9] In general, team-based care in diabetes is firmly rooted. The quality-improvement interventions with the greatest effect on improving glycemic control include adoption of multidisciplinary teams with expanded professional roles, non–medical record relay of information to physicians, and promotion of patient self-management.[28] Diabetes care teams involve primary care physicians, nurses, nurse educators, dietitians, and pharmacists but may expand to include endocrinologists, ophthalmologists, nephrologists, podiatrists, cardiologists, and vascular surgeons. Communication between care providers is an essential part of diabetes care.

Optimal glycemic control in patients with co-occurring HF and diabetes is unclear. Tighter glycemic control (A1c <6% vs 7%–8%) may increase mortality,[29] and this effect has also been observed in patients with HF.[30] The diabetes guidelines address the use of specific hypoglycemic agents in diabetic patients with HF.[31] Thiazolidinediones are contraindicated in symptomatic HF because of the associated peripheral edema and weight gain and should be used with caution in asymptomatic HF. US guidelines recommend that metformin be avoided in symptomatic HF or in the setting of renal insufficiency. However, based on observational data showing superior overall clinical outcomes in patients treated with metformin,[32,33] the European HF guidelines recommend metformin as the first-line therapy for the management of diabetes in patients with HF.[34] Limited data are available on the use of insulin and sulfonylureas in patients with HF. Meanwhile, there

are mechanistic reasons to think that the newer glucagon-like-peptide agents have intrinsic benefits in HF, though clinical trial data are not yet available. A clinical pharmacist can play a pivotal role in navigating the options for glycemic control in HF, considering drug-specific effects and side effects. In patients with more advanced HF, a dietitian may also be needed for the purpose of reconciling the protein-calorie nutritional needs of patients and their glycemic control.

Chronic Obstructive Pulmonary Disease

COPD is present in nearly one-third of patients with HF, with greater prevalence in HFpEF compared with HFrEF.[35] Treating HF in patients with COPD may be challenging, both because of the difficulty in distinguishing between cardiac and pulmonary causes of dyspnea and because of the need to balance beta-blockers in HF with beta-agonists in COPD. Although cardioselective beta-blockers (eg, metoprolol) have theoretic benefits over noncardioselective beta-blockers (eg, carvedilol) with regard to bronchoconstriction in patients with COPD, data are limited by the lack of enrollment of patients with known cardiovascular comorbidity in clinical trials of bronchodilators. In retrospective analysis, there was no evidence that beta-blocker cardioselectivity was associated with differences in outcomes for patients with HF with COPD versus those without.[36] For the long-term prevention of COPD exacerbations, the inhaled anticholinergic agent tiotropium is superior to the long-acting beta-2 agonist salmeterol[37]; however, a meta-analysis of inhaled anticholinergic trials demonstrated an increased risk of cardiovascular death, myocardial infarction, or stroke among patients with COPD using these agents.[38]

A team-based approach with pharmacist input and integration of pulmonary and cardiac diagnostic testing has much to offer in balancing the benefits and harms of pharmacotherapy in COPD and HF, but to date no such studies have been published. Limited literature on team-based care in COPD (using self-management, delivery system design, decision support, and clinical information systems) demonstrates lower rates of hospitalizations and emergency visits as well as shorter lengths of stay.[39] For patients with HF with COPD, an expanded care team including respiratory therapists, physical therapists, and exercise physiologists along with physiologic testing, such as ambulatory oxygen testing, pulmonary function testing, and cardiopulmonary stress testing, may help determine which condition is dominant in limiting exertion and causing dyspnea. Regardless of the dominant cause, many centers offer combined pulmonary and cardiac rehabilitation programs targeted at improvement of overall disability rather than a specific disease state; a combined approach has been demonstrated to be effective.[40]

Chronic Kidney Disease

HF and CKD interact bidirectionally to exacerbate one another in the cardiorenal syndrome.[41] CKD progression causes unfavorable changes in preload, afterload, inflammatory response, and hormonal systems, such as the renin-angiotensin-aldosterone system (RAAS) leading to worsening HF. Meanwhile, in patients with chronically or intermittently decompensated HF, the cycle of arterial hypoperfusion and especially venous congestion can lead to renal injury and progressive deterioration of renal function. Often the root cause of both HF and CKD are systemic illnesses: diabetes, hypertension, and other proinflammatory disease states. In these cases, team-based coordinated care across disciplines to manage diabetes, hypertension, lipids, and modify lifestyle is imperative. In patients with CKD, a multidisciplinary care team consisting of a nephrology nurse educator, renal dietitian, social worker, and pharmacy specialist, in addition to a nephrologist and vascular surgeon, can improve guideline adherence, slow the progression of renal disease, and improve overall survival.[42] In elderly patients with CKD, multidisciplinary care teams have been associated with reduced all-cause mortality and trends toward reduced hospitalization.[43]

The management of CKD in the setting of HF presents particular challenges regarding the use of diuretics. Worsening HF may result in diminished diuretic effectiveness, with diuretic braking and postdiuretic sodium retention, leading to a need for greater doses of diuretics.[44] Meanwhile, worsening renal function (WRF) is common in acute HF, occurring in 20% to 40% of patients.[45] However, even in advanced HF, it is the degree of venous congestion rather than the cardiac output that mediates worsening renal function[46]; congested patients with WRF often need more, not less, diuresis. Such decisions require knowledge of patient symptoms, volume status, and present renal function, achievable in hospitalized patients but challenging in nonhospitalized patients. In these instances, outpatient team-based care may preempt hospital admission and define the trajectory of cardiac and renal dysfunction. These teams may include nephrologists, HF cardiologists, HF nurses, primary care physicians, home care nurses, and dieticians. Discussions with patients with the severe HF and CKD may include consideration of advanced HF therapies, such as single-organ or combined-organ transplant and mechanical circulatory support.

RAAS blockers are fundamental in the therapy for HFrEF; but in moderate to advanced CKD, attention to serum potassium and creatinine clearance is required. Although prospective clinical trials to address the safety and effectiveness of RAAS blockade in patients with HF with CKD are lacking, propensity-matched analysis suggests that even in older patients with more advanced CKD (estimated glomerular filtration rate [eGFR] <45 mL/min/1.73 m^2), the prescription of RAAS blockade at discharge is associated with less hazard of death.[47] Guideline-based recommendations regarding renal dysfunction, potassium, and RAAS blockade are shown in **Table 3**. Navigating the changes in renal function and potassium with the use of RAAS blockers in HF and CKD requires care coordination between physician, nurse, pharmacist, and often home-care resources with iterative assessment of renal function, BP, and medication dosage.

Other Noncardiac Comorbidities

Osteoarthritis (OA) occurs in approximately 40% of patients with HF and may result in significant impairment in quality of life. Nonsteroidal antiinflammatory drugs (NSAIDs) are a foundation of therapy for OA, and those that preferentially inhibit cyclooxygenase-2 (COX-2) are less likely to cause gastrointestinal bleeding. However, COX-2–mediated increases in BP, sodium retention, and thrombosis worsen HF.[48] NSAID use is associated with the development of clinical HF[49–51] and increased mortality among those with a previous HF diagnosis.[52] Therapy for OA in HF is most safely achieved through avoidance of NSAIDs and specifically avoidance of COX-2–specific NSAIDs,[48] with a role for topical and nonpharmacologic (eg, physical therapy) approaches to pain relief.[53] A team approach with a primary care physician, nursing, pharmacy, physical and occupational therapy, and occasionally pain management specialists seems justified, though no literature currently exists to support such an intervention.

Cognitive impairment is present in up to 50% of patients with HF, and dementia occurs in about 25% of elderly patients with HF.[3] The co-occurrence of dementia and HF more than doubles hospital and home care costs compared with either condition alone.[54] In general, pharmacotherapy for HF may improve cognitive impairment in patients with HF[55]; exercise may also have salutary effects on cognition.[56] Multisource disease management programs for dementia

Table 3
Guideline-based recommendations regarding renal dysfunction, potassium, and RAAS blockade

Noncardiac Comorbidity	Therapeutic Considerations in Combined HF and Comorbidity	Team-Based Care Considerations	Pertinent Guidelines
CKD	ACE-inhibitor/angiotensin receptor blocker: caution if very low BPs (SBP <80 mm Hg), increased serum creatinine (>3 mg/dL), bilateral renal artery stenosis, elevated levels of serum potassium (>5.0 mEq/L) Aldosterone antagonists: serum creatinine <2.5 mg/dL (or eGFR >30 mL/min/1.73 m^2) and serum potassium <5.0 mEq/L without history of severe hyperkalemia	PCP, nephrologist, pharmacist, nurse coordinator, nutritionist	3,80
COPD	Cardioselective beta-blockers may cause less bronchoconstriction Inhaled anticholinergic agents may be superior to beta-agonists but associated with adverse cardiac events	PCP, pulmonologist, pharmacist, nurse coordinator Physical therapy, respiratory therapy	3,81
Diabetes Mellitus	Thiazolidinediones: predispose to edema, avoid in symptomatic HF Metformin: avoid in decompensated HF, renal failure; evidence overall in HF of improved outcomes GLP-1 receptor agonists: mechanistic rationale for benefit in HF, ongoing studies, limited guidance Dipeptidyl dipeptidase 4 inhibitors: associated with increased risk of HF, limited guidance Insulin: limited data on influence on HF outcomes Sulfonylureas: limited data on influence on HF outcomes	PCP, endocrinologist, pharmacist, nurse coordinator Diabetes educator, nutritionist, podiatrist, ophthalmologist	3,31,34
Hypertension	Consider class-specific effects In HFrEF prioritize ACE-inhibitor/angiotensin receptor blocker, beta-blocker, spironolactone; add hydralazine/nitrate in African Americans In HFpEF no agent proven to reduce mortality, major adverse cardiac events	PCP, pharmacist, nurse coordinator	3,19,20
Geriatrics	Avoid polypharmacy	PCP, geriatrician, pharmacist, nurse coordinator, home care, physical therapy	3,63
Osteoarthritis	Avoid NSAIDs (especially COX-2 specific)	PCP, rheumatologist, pharmacist, nurse coordinator, pain management	3,48,53
Dementia	Cholinesterase inhibitors modestly associated with bradycardia and hypotension	PCP, neurologist psychiatrist, psychologist, pharmacist, nurse coordinator	3,82
Depression	Uncertain effectiveness of SSRI in HF Role for regular exercise	PCP, psychiatrist, psychologist, pharmacist, nurse coordinator	3,83

Abbreviations: ACE, angiotensin-converting enzyme; COX-2, cyclooxygenase-2; GLP-1, glucagonlike peptide-1; NSAIDs, nonsteroidal antiinflammatory drugs; PCP, primary care physician; SBP, systolic BP; SSRI, selective serotonin reuptake inhibitor.

improve outcomes for both patients[57] and caregivers.[58] Whether team-based care strategies emphasizing effective pharmacologic and non-pharmacologic therapies in co-occurring HF and dementia can improve health care delivery and outcomes is not known.

Depression affects approximately 20% of patients with HF and is associated with increased mortality, hospitalization, and resource utilization.[59] Unfortunately, the largest trial of pharmacotherapy of depression in HF showed no improvement in either depression or cardiovascular status with the use of sertraline.[60] Structured aerobic exercise, however, may modestly improve depressive symptoms in HF.[61] Cognitive therapy may also be promising, but methodological variability limits the ability to apply existing evidence to real-world practice.[62] Whether multidisciplinary team-based approaches to HF and depression could synergize various therapeutic modalities for benefit remains to be seen.

Geriatric Care

The confluence of multiple comorbidities and the need to consider therapeutic trade-offs increases the need for flexibility and multidisciplinary approaches in geriatric patients.[63] Polypharmacy is a major issue in geriatrics, with studies showing that 44% of elderly patients discharged from an acute hospitalization are prescribed an inappropriate medication[64]; more than half of patients older than 65 years are receiving 5 or more medications[65]; and nearly 1 in 25 individuals are potentially at risk for a major drug-drug interaction.[66] Pharmacist-led interventions can have favorable effects on therapeutic, safety, hospitalization, and adherence outcomes in older adults[67]; inpatient geriatric specialty consultation to reduce errors in prescription or care transitions may have intermediate-term favorable effects on post-discharge outcomes.[68]

Although patients with HF with complex care needs are often in the geriatric age group, guidelines do not specify age-related contraindications to the use of medical or device-based therapies for HF. However, guidelines do recommend attention to eGFR as opposed to serum creatinine when considering angiotensin-converting enzyme inhibitors or angiotensin II receptor blockers caution regarding digoxin toxicity, and more frequent monitoring with more gradual changes during dose titration of guideline-directed medications in older patients.[3] As described elsewhere in this issue of Heart Failure Clinics, in patients with limited expected survival, the continued use of certain life-prolonging therapies, such as implantable cardioverter-defibrillators, should be revisited periodically as a patient ages or severity of illness progresses.

HEART FAILURE REHOSPITALIZATION AND THE ROLE OF NONCARDIAC COMORBIDITY

In the midst of an "epidemic of heart failure hospitalization,"[69] the impact of team-based care of noncardiac comorbidities on HF readmission rates is of great importance. Currently, readmission to the hospital within 30 days of HF hospital discharge occurs in 20% to 25% of patients and the associated costs are large, with Medicare shouldering approximately 45% of the burden.[70] Measures from Medicare penalizing hospitals with 30-day HF readmission rates in excess of a risk-standardized estimate have prompted the proliferation of programs geared toward readmission prevention, but preventing readmission after HF hospitalization is about more than HF. More than half of Medicare readmissions within 30 days of hospital discharge for HF are for non-HF diagnoses,[71] and such hospitalizations for noncardiovascular causes portend unfavorable long-term prognosis. In an analysis of the CHARM trial (Candesartan in Heart failure - Assessment of moRtality and Morbidity), though mortality within 30 days was greater after cardiovascular (CV) compared with non-CV hospitalization, subsequent rates of mortality were similar between CV and non-CV groups, a finding seen in both patients with HFrEF and patients with HFpEF.[72] Attention to comorbidity is a key to overall improvements in both survival and readmission, reflected in a recent transitional care trial involving an advanced practice nurse-directed discharge planning and home follow-up protocol. Readmissions and costs at 1 year were reduced, but the reduction in readmissions was primarily attributable to comorbidity-related readmissions, not HF-related readmissions, suggesting that multilevel interventions may improve care of comorbidities that drive readmissions.[73]

MULTIMORBIDITY

As described throughout this review, the management of comorbidities influences the delivery of care in HF. The presence of multiple comorbidities in HF can decrease patient self-efficacy and challenge self-care,[74] and chronic disease management of multiple comorbidities may exceed physician time available for patient care.[75] The impact of multiple interacting comorbidities may not be purely summative, particularly with the coexistence of 2 or more chronic conditions whereby neither condition is clearly dominant; this state has been termed *multimorbidity*.[76] A patient-centered approach focused on the overall multi-morbidity state in patients with HF may be most effective. As outlined by the American Geriatrics Society, this approach includes the following[77,78]:

- Elicitation or patient preferences
- Recognition of the limitations of applying the evidence base to a given individual
- Assessing prognosis and framing of risks and benefits with an emphasis on tradeoffs
- Recognizing therapeutic complexity and assessing feasibility
- Continual optimization of therapies to account for these factors and changes over time.

Multimorbidity interventions are emerging in the literature and tend to be complex and multifaceted with reorganization of care delivery and team-based approaches, resulting in modest improvements in prescribing and medication adherence with uncertain financial implications.[79] A large multisite intervention trial focusing on multimorbidity in HF is currently in development.

SUMMARY

HF is a condition in which the prognosis and treatment are often defined by comorbidities, many of which are noncardiac. Knowledge of the interactions between HF and specific comorbidities is essential, yet to date the clinical trial evidence base for managing comorbidity in patients with HF is limited; further investigations are clearly needed. Perhaps the most pressing need is a focus on the overall multimorbidity state and its relationship to HF—a need that should be addressed in forthcoming trials. Successful navigation between HF and common interacting comorbidities requires coordination of care and team-based approaches that continually evolve to meet patient needs.

REFERENCES

1. Go AS, Mozaffarian D, Roger VL, et al. Heart disease and stroke statistics–2014 update: a report from the American Heart Association. Circulation 2014;129(3):e28–292.
2. Heidenreich PA, Trogdon JG, Khavjou OA, et al. Forecasting the future of cardiovascular disease in the United States: a policy statement from the American Heart Association. Circulation 2011;123(8):933–44.
3. Yancy CW, Jessup M, Bozkurt B, et al. 2013 ACCF/AHA guideline for the management of heart failure: a report of the American College of Cardiology Foundation/American Heart Association Task Force on practice guidelines. Circulation 2013;128(16):e240–327.
4. Dall T, Blanchard T, Gallo P, et al. The economic impact of Medicare Part D on congestive heart failure. Am J Manag Care 2013;19:S97–100.
5. Braunstein JB, Anderson GF, Gerstenblith G, et al. Noncardiac comorbidity increases preventable hospitalizations and mortality among Medicare beneficiaries with chronic heart failure. J Am Coll Cardiol 2003;42(7):1226–33.
6. Wong CY, Chaudhry SI, Desai MM, et al. Trends in comorbidity, disability, and polypharmacy in heart failure. Am J Med 2011;124(2):136–43.
7. Ahluwalia SC, Gross CP, Chaudhry SI, et al. Change in comorbidity prevalence with advancing age among persons with heart failure. J Gen Intern Med 2011;26(10):1145–51.
8. van Deursen VM, Urso R, Laroche C, et al. Co-morbidities in patients with heart failure: an analysis of the European Heart Failure Pilot Survey. Eur J Heart Fail 2014;16:103–11.
9. Ahluwalia SC, Gross CP, Chaudhry SI, et al. Impact of comorbidity on mortality among older persons with advanced heart failure. J Gen Intern Med 2012;27(5):513–9.
10. Mentz RJ, Kelly JP, von Lueder TG, et al. Noncardiac comorbidities in heart failure with reduced versus preserved ejection fraction. J Am Coll Cardiol 2014;64(21):2281–93.
11. Lam CS, Donal E, Kraigher-Krainer E, et al. Epidemiology and clinical course of heart failure with preserved ejection fraction. Eur J Heart Fail 2011;13(1):18–28.
12. Bursi F, Weston S, Redfield M. Systolic and diastolic heart failure in the community. JAMA 2006;296(18):2209–16.
13. Bhatia R, Tu J, Lee D. Outcome of heart failure with preserved ejection fraction in a population-based study. N Engl J Med 2006;355(3):260–9.
14. Lenzen MJ, Scholte op Reimer WJ, Boersma E, et al. Differences between patients with a preserved and a depressed left ventricular function: a report from the EuroHeart Failure Survey. Eur Heart J 2004;25(14):1214–20.
15. Henkel DM, Redfield MM, Weston SA, et al. Death in heart failure: a community perspective. Circ Heart Fail 2008;1(2):91–7.
16. Ather S, Chan W, Bozkurt B, et al. Impact of noncardiac comorbidities on morbidity and mortality in a predominantly male population with heart failure and preserved versus reduced ejection fraction. J Am Coll Cardiol 2012;59(11):998–1005.
17. Mitchell P, Wynia M, Golden R, et al. Core principles & values of effective team-based health care. Discussion Paper, Institute of Medicine, Washington, DC. Available at: http://www.iom.edu/tbc.

18. Naylor M. Translational care: moving patients from one care setting to another. Am J Nurs 2009; 108(9 Suppl):58–63.

19. James PA, Oparil S, Carter BL, et al. 2014 evidence-based guideline for the management of high blood pressure in adults: report from the panel members appointed to the Eighth Joint National Committee (JNC 8). JAMA 2014;311(5):507–20.

20. Eckel RH, Jakicic JM, Ard JD, et al. 2013 AHA/ACC guideline on lifestyle management to reduce cardiovascular risk: a report of the American College of Cardiology/American Heart Association Task Force on Practice Guidelines. J Am Coll Cardiol 2014; 63(25 Pt B):2960–84.

21. Walsh J, McDonald K, Shojania K, et al. Quality improvement strategies for hypertension management: a systematic review. Med Care 2006;44(7): 646–57.

22. Carter BL, Rogers M, Daly J, et al. The potency of team-based care interventions for hypertension. Arch Intern Med 2009;169(19):1748–55.

23. Glynn LG, Murphy AW, Smith SM, et al. Interventions used to improve control of blood pressure in patients with hypertension. Cochrane Database Syst Rev 2010;(3):CD005182.

24. Martinez AS, Saef J, Paszczuk A, et al. Implementation of a pharmacist-managed heart failure medication titration clinic. Am J Health Syst Pharm 2013; 70(12):1070–6.

25. Steckler AE, Bishu K, Wassif H, et al. Telephone titration of heart failure medications. J Cardiovasc Nurs 2011;26(1):29–36.

26. Boudina S, Abel ED. Diabetic cardiomyopathy revisited. Circulation 2007;115(25):3213–23.

27. Iribarren C, Karter AJ, Go AS, et al. Clinical investigation and reports glycemic control and heart failure among adult patients with diabetes. Circulation 2001;103:2668–73.

28. Tricco AC, Ivers NM, Grimshaw JM, et al. Effectiveness of quality improvement strategies on the management of diabetes: a systematic review and meta-analysis. Lancet 2012;379(9833):2252–61.

29. Action to Control Cardiovascular Risk in Diabetes Study Group, Gerstein H, Miller ME, et al. Effects of intensive glucose lowering in type 2 diabetes. N Engl J Med 2008;358(24):2545–59.

30. Calles-Escandón J. Effect of intensive compared with standard glycemia treatment strategies on mortality by baseline subgroup characteristics the Action to Control Cardiovascular Risk in Diabetes (ACCORD) trial. Diabetes Care 2010;33(4): 721–7.

31. American Diabetes Association. Standards of medical care in diabetes–2014. Diabetes Care 2014; 37(Suppl 1):S14–80.

32. Masoudi FA, Inzucchi SE, Wang Y, et al. Thiazolidinediones, metformin, and outcomes in older patients with diabetes and heart failure: an observational study. Circulation 2005;111(5):583–90.

33. Eurich D, Majumdar S, McAlister FA, et al. Improved clinical outcomes associated with metformin in patients with diabetes and heart failure. Diabetes Care 2005;28(21):2345–51.

34. McMurray JJ, Adamopoulos S, Anker SD, et al. ESC guidelines for the diagnosis and treatment of acute and chronic heart failure 2012: the Task Force for the Diagnosis and Treatment of Acute and Chronic Heart Failure 2012 of the European Society of Cardiology. Developed in collaboration with the Heart Failure Association (HFA) of the ESC. Eur Heart J 2012; 33(14):1787–847.

35. Hawkins NM, Petrie MC, Jhund PS, et al. Heart failure and chronic obstructive pulmonary disease: diagnostic pitfalls and epidemiology. Eur J Heart Fail 2009;11(2):130–9.

36. Mentz RJ, Wojdyla D, Fiuzat M, et al. Association of beta-blocker use and selectivity with outcomes in patients with heart failure and chronic obstructive pulmonary disease (from OPTIMIZE-HF). Am J Cardiol 2013;111(4):582–7.

37. Vogelmeier C, Hederer B, Glaab T, et al. Tiotropium versus salmeterol for the prevention of exacerbations of COPD. N Engl J Med 2011;364(12): 1093–103.

38. Singh S, Loke Y, Furberg C. Inhaled anticholinergics and risk of major adverse cardiovascular events in patients with chronic obstructive pulmonary disease: a systematic review and meta-analysis. JAMA 2014;300(12):1439–50.

39. Adams S, Smith P. Systematic review of the chronic care model in chronic obstructive pulmonary disease prevention and management. Arch Intern Med 2007;167:551–61.

40. Evans RA, Singh SJ, Collier R, et al. Generic, symptom based, exercise rehabilitation; integrating patients with COPD and heart failure. Respir Med 2010;104(10):1473–81.

41. Ronco C, Haapio M, House AA, et al. Cardiorenal syndrome. J Am Coll Cardiol 2008;52(19):1527–39.

42. Chen Y-R, Yang Y, Wang S-C, et al. Effectiveness of multidisciplinary care for chronic kidney disease in Taiwan: a 3-year prospective cohort study. Nephrol Dial Transplant 2013;28(3):671–82.

43. Hemmelgarn BR, Manns BJ, Zhang J, et al. Association between multidisciplinary care and survival for elderly patients with chronic kidney disease. J Am Soc Nephrol 2007;18(3):993–9.

44. Ronco C, Cicoira M, McCullough PA. Cardiorenal syndrome type 1: pathophysiological crosstalk leading to combined heart and kidney dysfunction in the setting of acutely decompensated heart failure. J Am Coll Cardiol 2012;60(12):1031–42.

45. Butler J, Chirovsky D, Phatak H, et al. Renal function, health outcomes, and resource utilization in acute

heart failure: a systematic review. Circ Heart Fail 2010;3(6):726–45.

46. Mullens W, Abrahams Z, Francis GS, et al. Importance of venous congestion for worsening of renal function in advanced decompensated heart failure. J Am Coll Cardiol 2009;53(7):589–96.

47. Ahmed A, Fonarow GC, Zhang Y, et al. Renin-angiotensin inhibition in systolic heart failure and chronic kidney disease. Am J Med 2012;125(4):399–410.

48. Antman EM, Bennett JS, Daugherty A, et al. Use of nonsteroidal antiinflammatory drugs: an update for clinicians: a scientific statement from the American Heart Association. Circulation 2007;115(12):1634–42.

49. Feenstra J, Heerdink E, Grobbee D, et al. Association of nonsteroidal anti-inflammatory drugs with first occurrence of heart failure and with relapsing heart failure. Arch Intern Med 2014;162:265–70.

50. John P, David H. Consumption of NSAIDs and the development of congestive heart failure in elderly patients: an underrecognized public health problem. Arch Intern Med 2000;160:777–84.

51. Rodríguez L, Hernández-Díaz S. Nonsteroidal antiinflammatory drugs as a trigger of clinical heart failure. Epidemiology 2003;14:240–6.

52. Gislason G, Rasmussen J, Abildstrom S, et al. Increased mortality and cardiovascular morbidity associated with use of nonsteroidal anti-inflammatory drugs in chronic heart failure. Arch Intern Med 2009;169(2):141–9.

53. Hochberg MC, Altman RD, April KT, et al. American College of Rheumatology 2012 recommendations for the use of nonpharmacologic and pharmacologic therapies in osteoarthritis of the hand, hip, and knee. Arthritis Care Res (Hoboken) 2012; 64(4):465–74.

54. Maslow K. Dementia and serious coexisting medical conditions: a double whammy. Nurs Clin North Am 2004;39:561–79.

55. Dardiotis E, Giamouzis G, Mastrogiannis D, et al. Cognitive impairment in heart failure. Cardiol Res Pract 2012;2012:595821.

56. Gary RA, Brunn K. Aerobic exercise as an adjunct therapy for improving cognitive function in heart failure. Cardiol Res Pract 2014;2014:157508.

57. Vickrey B, Mittman B, Connor K, et al. The effect of a disease management intervention on quality and outcomes in dementia care. Ann Intern Med 2006; 145(10):727.

58. Belle S, Burgio L, Burns R, et al. Enhancing the quality of life of dementia caregivers from different ethnic or racial groups. Ann Intern Med 2006;145:727–38.

59. Rutledge T, Reis VA, Linke SE, et al. Depression in heart failure a meta-analytic review of prevalence, intervention effects, and associations with clinical outcomes. J Am Coll Cardiol 2006;48(8):1527–37.

60. O'Connor CM, Jiang W, Kuchibhatla M, et al. Safety and efficacy of sertraline for depression in patients with heart failure: results of the SADHART-CHF (Sertraline Against Depression and Heart Disease in Chronic Heart Failure) trial. J Am Coll Cardiol 2010; 56(9):692–9.

61. Blumenthal JA, Babyak MA, Connor CO, et al. Effects of exercise training on depressive symptoms in patients with chronic heart failure. JAMA 2014; 308(5):465–74.

62. Dekker R. Cognitive therapy for depression in patients with heart failure: a critical review. Heart Fail Clin 2012;43(1):127–41.

63. Partnership for Health in Aging Workgroup on Interdisciplinary Team Training in Geriatrics. Position statement on interdisciplinary team training in geriatrics: an essential component of quality health care for older adults. J Am Geriatr Soc 2014;62(5):961–5.

64. Hajjar E, Cafiero A, Hanlon J. Polypharmacy in elderly patients. Am J Geriatr Pharmacother 2007; 5(4):345–51.

65. Kaufman DW, Kelly JP, Rosenberg L, et al. Recent patterns of medication use in the ambulatory adult population of the United States. JAMA 2014; 287(3):337–44.

66. Qato D, Alexander G, Conti R. Use of prescription and over-the-counter medications and dietary supplements among older adults in the United States. JAMA 2008;300(24):2867–78.

67. Lee JK, Slack MK, Martin J, et al. Geriatric patient care by U.S. pharmacists in healthcare teams: systematic review and meta-analyses. J Am Geriatr Soc 2013;61(7):1119–27.

68. Deschodt M, Flamaing J, Haentjens P, et al. Impact of geriatric consultation teams on clinical outcome in acute hospitals: a systematic review and meta-analysis. BMC Med 2013;11(1):48.

69. Giamouzis G, Kalogeropoulos A, Georgiopoulou V, et al. Hospitalization epidemic in patients with heart failure: risk factors, risk prediction, knowledge gaps, and future directions. J Card Fail 2011; 17(1):54–75.

70. Pfuntner A, Wier LM, Steiner C. Costs for Hospital Stays in the United States, 2010. HCUP Statistical brief # 146. 2013. Agency for Healthcare Research and Quality, Rockville, MD. Available at: http://www.hcup-us.ahrq.gov/reports/statbriefs/sb146.pdf.

71. Dharmarajan K, Hsieh A, Lin Z, et al. Diagnoses and timing of 30-day readmissions after hospitalization for heart failure, acute myocardial infarction, or pneumonia. JAMA 2013;309(4):355–63.

72. Desai AS, Claggett B, Pfeffer MA, et al. Influence of hospitalization for cardiovascular versus noncardiovascular reasons on subsequent mortality in patients with chronic heart failure across the spectrum of ejection fraction. Circ Heart Fail 2014; 7(6):895–902.

73. Naylor M, Brooten D, Campbell RL, et al. Transitional care of older adults hospitalized with heart failure: a

randomized, controlled trial. J Am Geriatr Soc 2004; 52:675–84.

74. Dickson VV, Buck H, Riegel B. Multiple comorbid conditions challenge heart failure self-care by decreasing self-efficacy. Nurs Res 2013;62(1):2–9.

75. Østbye T, Yarnall K, Krause K, et al. Is there time for management of patients with chronic diseases in primary care? Ann Fam Med 2005;3:209–14.

76. Boyd CM, Fortin M. Future of multimorbidity research: how should understanding of multimorbidity inform health system design. Public Health Rev 2011;32(2):451–74.

77. American Geriatrics Society Expert Panel on the Care of Older Adults with Multimorbidity. Patient-centered care for older adults with multiple chronic conditions: a stepwise approach from the American Geriatrics Society: American Geriatrics Society Expert Panel on the Care of Older Adults with Multimorbidity. J Am Geriatr Soc 2012;60(10):1957–68.

78. Guiding principles for the care of older adults with multimorbidity: an approach for clinicians. Guiding principles for the care of older adults with multimorbidity: an approach for clinicians: American Geriatrics Society Expert Panel on the Care of Older Adults with Multimorbidity. J Am Geriatr Soc 2012; 60(10):E1–25.

79. Sm S, Soubhi H, Fortin M, et al. Interventions for improving outcomes in patients with multimorbidity in primary care and community settings [review]. Cochrane Database Syst Rev 2013;(4):CD006560.

80. Drüeke TB, Parfrey PS. Summary of the KDIGO guideline on anemia and comment: reading between the guidelines. Kidney Int 2012;82(9):952–60. Available at: http://kdigo.org/home/guidelines/.

81. Qaseem A, Wilt TJ, Weinberger SE, et al. Clinical guideline diagnosis and management of stable chronic obstructive pulmonary disease: a clinical practice guideline update from the American College of Physicians, American College of Chest Physicians, American Thoracic Society, and European Respiratory Society. Ann Intern Med 2011;155:179–92.

82. Qaseem A, Snow V, Cross JT Jr, et al. Current pharmacologic treatment of dementia: a clinical practice guideline. Ann Intern Med 2007;148:370–8.

83. Gelenberg AJ, Freeman MP, Markowitz JC, et al. Practice guideline for the treatment of patients with major depressive disorder. 3rd edition. Arlington, VA: American Psychiatric Association; 2010.

Team-based Care for Cardiac Rehabilitation and Exercise Training in Heart Failure

Bunny Pozehl, PhD, APRN-NP[a],*, Rita McGuire, PhD, RN[b], Joseph Norman, PhD, PT[c]

KEYWORDS

- Heart failure • Cardiac rehabilitation • Exercise training • Heart failure–reduced ejection fraction
- Heart failure–preserved ejection fraction

KEY POINTS

- Cardiac rehabilitation (CR) for heart failure (HF) -reduced ejection fraction is now reimbursed by the Centers for Medicare and Medicaid. Many major insurance companies also reimburse CR irrespective of type or severity of HF.
- Current guidelines of care for HF recommend exercise; however, specifics of appropriate exercise training are not detailed.
- Components of traditional CR do not currently include HF disease management. A few resources do outline recommendations for CR in patients with HF.
- The American Association of Cardiovascular and Pulmonary Rehabilitation has outlined core competencies for CR and secondary prevention professionals and a team of multidisciplinary providers is needed to collectively meet core competency recommendations for delivery of CR.
- Addition of a HF disease management component to CR would necessitate that providers with HF expertise be included as team members to assist in the management of the patient with HF participating in CR.

Cardiac rehabilitation (CR) has long been an effective secondary prevention intervention for eligible patients with known cardiovascular disease. Patients with heart failure (HF) however have not been eligible for reimbursement of CR services until recently. This lack of reimbursement was a reflection of the state of the science or lack of evidence related to exercise training in HF. Before the large multicenter HF-ACTION (Heart Failure–A Controlled Trial Investigating Outcomes of Exercise Training)[1] trial, the benefits of exercise training for patients with HF and reduced ejection fraction (HFrEF) had only been documented in numerous small studies.[2] As a result of the collective body of evidence and the established safety of exercise in patients with stable chronic HFrEF, the Centers for Medicare and Medicaid (CMS) extended coverage for patients with HFrEF in 2014. Research data are much more limited to date on the effects of exercise training for patients with HF and preserved ejection fraction (HFpEF),[3–9] and therefore, there is no current CMS approval for reimbursement of CR in these patients. In addition to CMS coverage, a recent survey of large commercial health care insurance companies in the United States showed that 29 of 44 (66%) provided coverage for outpatient CR for patients with HF.[10] Interestingly, 24 of these 29 companies provided coverage irrespective of the type

[a] University of Nebraska Medical Center, College of Nursing, 1230 O Street, Suite 131, Lincoln, NE 68588-0220, USA; [b] University of Nebraska Medical Center, College of Nursing, 1230 O Street, Suite 131, Lincoln, NE 68588-0220, USA; [c] Division of Physical Therapy Education, 984420 Nebraska Medical Center, Omaha, NE 68198-4420, USA
* Corresponding author.
E-mail address: bpozehl@unmc.edu

Heart Failure Clin 11 (2015) 431–449
http://dx.doi.org/10.1016/j.hfc.2015.03.007
1551-7136/15/$ – see front matter © 2015 Elsevier Inc. All rights reserved.

or severity of HF.[10] Clearly, the landscape of exercise training and CR in patients with HF is expanding and evolving. It is important to consider the implications this has for the team-based care required to deliver these services to this patient population.

HEART FAILURE GUIDELINES ADDRESSING EXERCISE IN HEART FAILURE

It is important to review the current care management guidelines for HF and to consider what these guidelines provide in terms of recommendations for exercise in the patient with HF (**Table 1**). The guidelines reviewed recommended physical activity[11,12] or exercise[13–15] for HF patients (Level of evidence I A). Terms associated with exercise included "regular"[11,13] and "moderate daily activity."[12] Only one guideline specified time and intensity of exercise: 30 minutes of moderate-intensity exercise 5 days per week with warm-up and cool-down exercises[14] (Strength of Evidence B), and one stated the uncertainty of an optimal exercise "prescription."[13] Exercise training is recommended for HF patients[11–15] as safe and effective to improve functional status[11] (Level of Evidence A). Of note is the recommendation from the Heart Failure Society of America[13] for exercise testing to determine suitability/safety of exercise training.[14] Specifics related to exercise training included facilitating the understanding of heart rate ranges, appropriate levels of exercise training, and other exercise expectations.[14] Exercise training should include increasing duration and intensity of exercise in a supervised setting and promotion of adherence to training.[14] Cardiac rehabilitation[11]/supervised group-based exercise[14,15] was specifically recommended for those with stable chronic HF[11,12,15] (Level of Evidence B) with no precluding heart conditions or devices.[15] Lainscak and colleagues[12] reported there was no evidence limiting exercise training to any particular subgroup of HF patients. Overall, the HF guidelines provide limited detail on the specifics of exercise training for HF patients.[11–16]

Table 1
Exercise recommendations from general guidelines of care in heart failure

Reference	Recommendation
AACVPR,[16] 2014	Physician-prescribed exercise: Exercise training and other therapeutic exercise, including aerobic and strength training
McMurray et al,[14] 2012	Regular aerobic exercise to improve functional capacity and symptoms [I A]

Lindenfeld et al,[13] 2010	• Exercise testing to determine suitability for exercise training (patient does not develop significant ischemia or arrhythmias) (strength of evidence = B)
	• If deemed safe, exercise training should be considered:
	  ○ To facilitate understanding of exercise expectations
	  ○ To increase exercise duration and intensity
	  ○ In a supervised setting
	  ○ To promote adherence
	  ○ Exercise goal of 30 min of moderate activity/exercise, 5 d/wk with warm-up and cool-down exercises (strength of evidence = B)

Yancy et al,[11] 2013	Activity, exercise prescription, and CR recommendations:
	Class I
	  Exercise training (or regular physical activity) is recommended as safe and effective for patients with HF who are able to participate to improve functional status (level of evidence = A)
	Class IIa
	  CR can be useful in clinically stable patient with HF to improve functional capacity, exercise duration, health-related quality of life, and mortality (level of evidence = B)

Lainscak et al,[12] 2011	Current guidelines • Regular moderate daily activity • Exercise training if available
National Institute for Health and Care Excellence,[15] 2014	Stable chronic HF and no precluding condition or device offered a supervised group exercise-based CR program that includes education and psychological support

Adapted from Refs.[11–16]

CURRENT EXERCISE TRAINING GUIDELINES AND POSITION STATEMENTS FOR PATIENTS WITH HEART FAILURE

As illustrated in the review of HF guidelines, there is a lack of detail concerning specifics of exercise training in HF; therefore, it is important to review what is specified in available position statements and guidelines that are specific for exercise training in HF. Four official exercise-training position statements or guidelines were found in the literature (**Table 2**).[17–20] Several additional references presented by individual authors provide helpful principles and guidelines for implementation of exercise training in HF.[21–26] Systematic reviews and meta-analyses also provide helpful summaries of exercise training and patient outcomes for patients with HF.[2,27–32] Two exercise-training guidelines specify absolute contraindications to exercise testing and training for patients with HF, and these should be considered with thorough evaluation of the patient before participation in exercise training (**Table 3**).[18,20] Relative contraindications are predominately symptomatic responses, such as increased weight, blood pressure, heart rate, or arrhythmias, that are clinical indicators of instability that may place the patient at increased risk with exercise. Consideration of absolute and relative contraindications is essential to insure safety of the patient for exercise training in HF.[17–20]

There are many commonalities in exercise-training protocols across the guideline statements in terms of mode or type, frequency, intensity, and duration of exercise.[17–20] The type or mode of exercise specifies aerobic in all statements with a recommendation for consideration of steady state or intermittent/intervals of rest and exercise as needed for deconditioned patients. Aerobic exercise included use of machines (eg, treadmill, cycle ergometer, step and rowing machines) in addition to calisthenics and walking. Three of the most recent statements included specific details for resistance training with training outlined for different New York Heart Association (NYHA) classes or use of a staged approach to this training.[17,18,20] The earliest guideline from Pina and colleagues[19] stated that the safety and efficacy of resistive training had not been established but noted that small free weights, elastic bands, or repetitive isolated muscle training may be used. The European guideline also presented respiratory training, especially for those individuals with inspiratory muscle weakness.[18]

Frequency of exercise ranged across the guidelines from 3 to 7 days per week with 3 to 5 days per week being most common. Intensity ranges from 40% to 80% Vo_{2peak} and emphasized starting at a lower intensity in the deconditioned. Progression to 80% Vo_{2peak} exercise should be in hospitals or centers with advanced cardiac life support (ACLS) -trained individuals. Intensity was presented as rating of perceived exertion (RPE) with a range of 9 to 14 on a Borg scale of 6 to 20 being acceptable. Duration of exercise is emphasized starting with 5 to 10 minutes and progressing up to 20 to 60 minutes per session. Warm-up and cool-down were advised.[17–20]

In summary, the guidelines and position statements for exercise in HF provided specific guidance for mode or type, frequency, intensity, and duration of exercise. What was not presented in these guidelines was a discussion of team-based management to implement exercise training. Determination of suitability of the patient to safely exercise obviously requires assessment and evaluation by a medical provider and preferably that provider should be a cardiologist or HF specialist. Implementation of the exercise-training protocol and evaluation of patient response clearly requires the expertise of an exercise specialist. No additional team members were discussed or implied in this review of the guidelines and position statements for exercise in HF. Consideration for additional team members was much more obvious in guidelines related to CR.

COMPONENTS OF TRADITIONAL CARDIAC REHABILITATION

CR and secondary prevention programs serve an integral role in the comprehensive management of individuals with cardiovascular disorders.[33,34] These programs were based on effective, evidence-based interventions and strategies to optimize health, lifestyle, and quality of life of individuals with heart disease. Consensus statements and guidelines from major professional associations (American Heart Association [AHA], American College of Cardiology [ACC], American Association of Cardiovascular and Pulmonary Rehabilitation [AACVPR], Agency for Health Care Policy and Research, European Society of Cardiology [ESC], and British Association for Cardiovascular Prevention and Rehabilitation)[33–38] recommend a comprehensive, interprofessional approach to address cardiovascular risk and physical conditioning. The broad areas that need to be encompassed in the overall management scheme of individuals in CR/secondary prevention programs were as follows: (1) baseline patient assessment; (2) nutritional counseling and cardiovascular risk factor management; (3) psychosocial interventions; and (4) physical activity counseling and exercise training.[33,34] To this end, there exists a high degree of consistency across organizations regarding the core

Table 2
Exercise training in heart failure—position statements and guidelines

		Reference
Adsett & Mullins,[17] 2014	Considerations	Comprehensive assessment of patient to stratify risk
	Mode	Steady state or intermittent/interval; cycle ergometer, treadmill, rowing machines, step aerobics, calisthenics; swimming and Tai Chi also discussed
	Frequency	Tailor frequency to each individual: minimum 3–5 d/wk
	Intensity	50%–70% Vo_{2peak} or 60%–80% heart rate reserve; RPE between 9 and 14 on the Borg 6–20 scale
	Duration	Start at short durations 10–20 min and progress to longer sessions 30–40 min
	Resistance training	Avoid isometric exercises Intensity: Light weights only; workload of 40% One-repetition maximum (1 RM) progress to 60% 1 RM; 9–13 on RPE (6–20) Repetitions and sets: 8–15 repetitions; 2–4 sets Frequency: 1–2 d/wk Duration: 20–30 min
Piepoli et al,[18] 2011	Considerations	Patient selection and functional examination: Medical history, clinical examination, resting electrocardiogram, symptom-limited exercise test, echocardiography Individualized prescription
	Mode	Calisthenic exercises or gentle individualized gradual mobilization for severe HF patients with physical deconditioning, cachexia, or other recent clinical instability Endurance aerobic (continuous and interval); resistance/strength; respiratory training
	Frequency	3–5 d/wk; start twice weekly in deconditioned
	Intensity	Start at 40%–50%, increase to 70%–80% Vo_{2peak}; RPE <15
	Duration	Start 5–10 min and progress to 20–60 min
	Resistance training	3 stages for resistance training: 1. Pretraining: Intensity <30% 1 RM; RPE <12; 5–10 repetitions; 2–3 sessions per wk, 1–3 circuits each session 2. Resistance/endurance training: Intensity 30%–40% 1 RM: RPE 12–13; repetitions 12–25; 2–3 sessions per wk; 1 circuit per session 3. Strength training/muscle building: Intensity 40%–60% 1 RM; RPE <15; 8–15 repetitions; 2–3 sessions per wk; 1 circuit per session Avoid Valsalva or abdominal straining; should be able to perform 10 repetitions
	Respiratory training	Intensity: Start at 30% of inspiratory mouth pressure and readjust intensity every 7–10 d up to a maximum of 60% Frequency: 3–5 sessions per wk Duration: Minimum 8 wk
Pina et al,[19] 2003	Considerations	Assessment of functional capacity; no agreement on universal exercise prescription; individualized approach recommended
	Mode	Most commonly treadmill and bicycle ergometry May need to consider intervals of rest
	Frequency	3–5 d/wk Supplemental walking on nontraining days
	Intensity	70%–80% peak Vo_2; 60%–65% peak Vo_2 and interval training with periods of rest in very debilitated patients Borg scale RPE of 12–13
	Duration	Adequate warm-up of 10–15 min (longer in debilitated patients) 20–30 min at desired intensity Cool-down advised
	Resistance training	Safety and efficacy of resistive training has not been established Small free weights (1, 2, or 5 lb), elastic bands, or repetitive isolated muscle training may be used

(continued on next page)

Table 2		
(continued)		

		Reference
Selig et al,[20] 2010	Considerations	Stable patient as determined by medical practitioner; symptom-limited exercise and functional testing prior; tailored program to meet individual's functional and symptomatic status
	Mode	Aerobic training
		Interval training initially 1:1 exercise/rest ratio progressing to 2:1 exercise/rest ratio
	Frequency	4–7 d/wk
	Intensity	NYHA class I–II
		40%–75% of HR_{peak} or 40%–70% of Vo_{2peak}, up to 80% Vo_{2peak} if applied in hospitals or centers with ACLS-trained personnel
		RPE 11–14 (Borg 6–20 point scale)
		NYHA class III-IV
		40%–65% HR_{peak} where HR_{peak} is predetermined in a symptom-limited graded exercise test or 40%–60% Vo_{2peak}
		RPE ≤ 13
	Duration	Commence at 10–15 min at target exercise intensity, progress gradually to 45–60 min based on tolerance
	Resistance training	Resistance training (circuit weight-training, TheraBand exercise, body weight exercise) 2–3 d/wk
		NYHA class I–II
		6–15 repetitions per set;4–8 different exercises for major muscle groups; commence at 1 set per exercise progress to 3 sets; RPE 11–14 (Borg 6–20 point scale)
		NYHA class III-IV
		4–10 repetitions per set; 3–4 different exercises for major muscle groups; commence at 1 set per exercise progress to 2 sets; RPE 10–13 (Borg 6–20 point scale)
		Flexibility 2–3 d/wk; 5–10 min; stretch the major muscle groups affecting the hips, knees, upper and lower spine, chest, and shoulders

Adapted from Refs.[17–20]

components that need to be included in a comprehensive CR/secondary prevention program (**Table 4**). The recommendations and guidelines across organizations were closely aligned as were the targeted treatment goals. There was a slight difference between the American[39] and European[36] guidelines for the lower cut point used to determine impaired fasting glycemia (≥ 5.6 mmol vs 6.1–6.9 mmol, respectively), but otherwise, close agreement exists on the management of diabetes as well as the other core components.

RECOMMENDATIONS FOR CARDIAC REHABILITATION IN PATIENTS WITH HEART FAILURE

Literature that specifically addressed CR for patients with HF included one regulatory statement from CMS,[45] one position statement from Working Group on Cardiac Rehabilitation and Exercise Physiology of the ESC,[46] and 4 additional articles targeting CR for HF (**Table 5**).[47–50]

Although each of these references included exercise training, they were much more broadly focused on essential elements of care management required for patients with HF in a CR setting.

Common components included exercise training, psychosocial assessment, support and counseling, outcomes assessment, and education.[45–50] The regulatory statement from CMS mirrored regular CR without a discussion of HF-specific care management.[45] The ESC statement clearly identified 6 core components that include specific HF care management. In the ESC statement, CR was described as a continuum of services that spanned inpatient and outpatient settings and should be available to every eligible HF patient.[46] A multidisciplinary team comprising a cardiologist, a designated program coordinator, and other team members with needed expertise was the recommended model for CR.[46]

The remaining 4 articles that discussed CR for patients with HF emphasized the need to incorporate education and guidance with self-care

Table 3
Contraindications to exercise testing and training in heart failure

Absolute Contraindications to Exercise Testing and Training	Relative Contraindications or Increased Risk for Exercise Training
• Progressive worsening of exercise tolerance or dyspnea over previous 3–5 d[18,20] • Significant ischemia at low exercise intensity (<2 metabolic equivalent of task (METS) or ~50 Watts)[18,20] • Uncontrolled diabetes[18,20] • Recent embolism[18,20] • Thrombophlebitis[18,20] • Acute systemic illness or fever[18,20] • Acute myocarditis and pericarditis[18,20] • Symptomatic aortic stenosis[18] • Severe aortic stenosis[20] • Severe hypertrophic obstructive cardiomyopathy[18] • Intracardiac thrombus[18] • Early phase after acute coronary syndrome (up to 2 d)[18] • Untreated life-threatening cardiac arrhythmias[18] • Acute HF with hemodynamic instability[18] • Uncontrolled hypertension[18] • Advanced atrioventricular block[18] • Regurgitant valvular heart disease requiring surgery[20] • Myocardial infarction within previous 3 wk[20] • New onset atrial fibrillation/atrial flutter[18,20] • Resting heart rate >120 bpm[20]	• >1.8 kg increase in body mass over the previous 1–3 d[18] • >2 kg increase in body mass over previous 1–3 d[20] • Concurrent, continuous, or intermittent dobutamine therapy[18,20] • Decrease in systolic blood pressure with exercise[18,20] • NYHA functional class IV[18,20] • Complex ventricular arrhythmia at rest or appearing with exertion[18,20] • Supine resting heart rate >100 bpm[18,20] • Pre-existing comorbidities limiting exercise tolerance[18,20] • Moderate aortic stenosis[20] • BP >180/110 mm Hg (evaluate on case-by-case basis)

behaviors essential to HF management; this goes above and beyond what has traditionally been provided for education and guidance in CR programs. It necessitates multidisciplinary team members that have HF management expertise.[47–50]

REFERRAL AND PARTICIPATION IN CARDIAC REHABILITATION

CR is currently underused in both the United States and Europe for all cardiac patients. Pack and colleagues[51] report that CR utilization in the United States was 28% of eligible patients with cardiovascular disease. A similar percentage (28.5%) was reported for participation in the United Kingdom.[52] These numbers referred to all cardiac patients eligible for CR and not just patients with HF. Bjarnason-Wehrens and colleagues[53] examined CR attendance by patients with HF in Europe and found less than 20% attend. Many factors have been identified that contribute to underutilization of CR services. The 2010 Update from the AACVPR and the ACA Foundation/AHA Task Force on Performance Measures for Cardiac Rehabilitation[54] identified patient-oriented factors, medical factors

(previously provider-oriented barriers), and health care system factors that should be addressed in relation to CR referral and participation. These performance measures pointed to specific areas that the team responsible for delivery of CR or exercise training needs to focus on to improve care and increase referral and participation to CR services.

Literature-reporting barriers or factors that impacted exercise in patients with HF are summarized in **Table 6**.[18,55–59] These barriers or factors can be organized in a manner similar to the Performance Measures on Cardiac Rehabilitation (ie, patient-oriented, medical or provider oriented, and health care system factors) created by Thomas and colleagues.[54] Patient level barriers included common barriers to exercise noted by healthy individuals, such as lack of time, lack of motivation, attitude toward exercise, financial constraints, transportation issues, inclement weather, depression, and older age. In addition to these common barriers, patients with HF had unique barriers to exercise that stemmed from the chronic illness of HF, including fear of overdoing, lack of energy, symptoms (shortness of breath), cognitive issues, and lack of insight into benefits of exercise.[18,55,57–59] These unique barriers pointed to a need to consider the knowledge, skills, and confidence that may be lacking for patients with HF to self-manage exercise behavior. As previously stated, a relative contraindication to exercise that may put patients with HF at increased risk was a 1.8- or 2-kg increase in weight over the previous 1 to 3 days.[18,20] Patients who are active and engaged in self-management behavior for HF may already know the importance of daily weights and monitoring symptoms; however, this must have even greater emphasis if engaging in routine exercise. Accomplishing behavior change such as exercise requires that patients assume self-management responsibility. Practical guidelines for self-care management of HF (eg, the position statement by Lainscak and colleagues[12] from the ESC) may be helpful to providers and team members trying to promote self-management behavior in HF.

Typical system level issues that may serve as barriers to CR participation included lack of referral; lack of exercise sites/programs; and lack of resources (eg, support, HF-trained personnel, and reimbursement).[18,55,57,58] System level factors are quite significant considering the Pack and colleagues[51] report of current and potential capacity for CR utilization in the United States. This report estimates that a maximum of 47% of qualifying patients in the United States could be serviced by existing programs even with modest expansion of all existing programs. Current program directors reported feeling limited by facilities, personnel, and copays/insurance problems rather than patient behavior.[51] These authors concluded that currently there is insufficient capacity to meet national service needs, and they called for alternative models of delivery, such as group-based CR programs in community centers, home-based programs, and Web-based methods of delivering CR. Implications for the team responsible for CR in patients with HF are significant given that current CR programs may not be prepared or educated in the specific care management that has been outlined for delivery of CR in patients with HF. Conraads and colleagues,[57] in the 2012 ESC position statement, noted that there is limited availability of rehabilitation programs or exercise facilities that were suitable for patients with HF. The Presidential Advisory from the AHA by Balady and colleagues[55] concerning referral, enrollment, and delivery of CR programs, set out policy recommendations and discussed opportunities to expand CR services through health reform implementation. It will be critical that providers who are familiar with care management of patients with HF be involved in decisions related to future policies and health care reform implementation

for CR to meet the needs of patients with HF and provide quality care in the health care reform era.

Finally, the provider-oriented barriers or medical factors that contributed to lack of participation of patients with HF in CR or exercise training must be considered. The science underlying safe and beneficial exercise in stable chronic HF must be presented to providers to educate and perhaps change perspectives and beliefs concerning the need and benefit of patients participating in CR or exercise training. Many HF providers never mentioned exercise,[58] and less than 60% of cardiac patients eligible for CR were actually referred for participation.[60] Providers must recognize exercise training and CR as an important nonpharmacologic intervention that can benefit the stable chronic HF patient.

RESOURCE CONSIDERATIONS FOR TEAM-BASED CARDIAC REHABILITATION AND EXERCISE TRAINING FOR HEART FAILURE

Medical directors of CR programs are responsible for the delivery of safe, effective, and high-quality services to eligible patients.[61] The 2012 AACVPR/AHA Scientific Statement concerning medical director responsibilities for outpatient CR programs outlined 6 broad categories of responsibility, including: (1) supervision of qualified multidisciplinary staff; (2) referral and enrollment of appropriate patients; (3) oversight of the Individualized Treatment Plan; (4) directing progress of individual patients; (5) education of patients and health care professionals; and (6) outcomes assessment.[61] Regulatory requirements by CMS of the physician responsible for a CR program included expertise in the management of individuals with cardiac physiology. Cardiac expertise would be invaluable in directing CR care for patients with HF. The medical director could educate both patients and staff in the unique needs and concerns for the patient with HF. The role of the medical director as a team leader was discussed as a core concept that is especially critical in changing health care delivery models with emphasis on patient-centered outcomes and cost-effective care.

Obviously, the medical director of a CR program must collaborate effectively with a qualified multidisciplinary staff in the delivery of team-based care. In the 2012 Science Advisory from the AHA, Arena and colleagues[62] addressed the valuable role of health care professionals in inpatient and home health settings to encourage referral and participation in CR. This document actually identified specific team members, including nursing, physical therapy, clinical exercise physiologists, registered dieticians, and physicians, who are key

Table 4
Summary of cardiac rehabilitation/secondary prevention program core components for all cardiovascular disorders

Core Components	Patient-Centered Medical Care and Management
Patient assessment	Evaluation: Physical examination, medical history (including comorbidities and symptom assessment), 12-lead resting electrocardiogram, postprocedure, laboratory tests, imaging studies, cardiovascular risk profile, education barriers and preferences, assess medications, influenza vaccination status, patient's perceived health status and quality of life, assess functional status Intervention: Monitor effectiveness of pharmacotherapy (adjust as indicated), compliance with medications, assessment of medical control/stability, develop an individualized treatment plan using the other core components to address physical health and psychosocial well-being/cardiovascular risk factor reduction/improved symptom management/greater level of physical activity and exercise/enhanced quality of life, arrange for patient to have annual influenza vaccination Expected outcomes: Medical stability, management of symptoms, establish short-term and long-term goals, discharge plan
Nutritional counseling	Evaluation: Assess total daily caloric intake and dietary content (saturated fats, trans fat, cholesterol, sodium, nutrients), evaluate eating habits and patterns, identify areas needing specific dietary intervention to address other core components as well as comorbidities Interventions: Prescribe and tailor specific recommendations for a cardioprotective diet, educate and counsel patient and associated caregivers and family, provide education on self-monitoring of weight, edema, and symptoms, the individualized dietary modification plan should be sensitive to personal and cultural variables Expected outcomes: Compliant with dietary recommendations, plan established to address eating behaviors or problems, patient knowledgeable about appropriate dietary content, portions, and relapse prevention/management
Weight management	Evaluation: Measure height, weight, calculate body mass index, obtain waist circumference Interventions: Establish reasonable, individualized goals to reduce weight, develop a reduced calorie dietary plan in conjunction with a physical activity/exercise program and behavioral modification program, tailor programs to the individual to reduce body weight, use pharmacotherapy if appropriate, educate patient on relapse management Expected outcomes: Establish short-term goals to achieve a progressive loss of weight, establish long-term goals for attaining desired weight and maintenance of desired weight goal, patient knowledgeable in relapse prevention/management

Blood pressure management	**Evaluation:** Measurements of seated blood pressure on multiple visits, measurements taken/compared in both arms, and in various positions (lying, seated, standing) to assess for orthostatic hypotension, assess current medication regime effectiveness and patient adherence, assess for nonprescription drugs being taken that may adversely impact blood pressure **Interventions:** Monitor blood pressure at rest and during physical activity/exercise, advise/educate on lifestyle modifications (physical activity/ exercise, weight management, moderate sodium restriction, dietary intake, alcohol moderation, tobacco cessation) to assist in managing blood pressure, initiate/monitor pharmacotherapy, following the guidelines in the Joint National Committee (JNC) 7 report guidelines[40] **Expected outcomes:** Blood pressure maintained at goal level, patient adherent to prescribed medications and lifestyle modification strategies
Lipid management	**Evaluation:** Fasting lipid profile (total cholesterol, high-density lipoprotein, low-density lipoprotein, and triglycerides), obtain history of diet, medications, and comorbidities that may impact lipid levels, assess current treatment strategies and patient adherence, reassessment of lipid profile 4–6 wk after hospitalization or 2 mo after initiation of interventions, assessment based on using National Cholesterol Education Program (NCEP)-Adult Treatment Panel (ATP) III guidelines[41,42] **Interventions:** Provide dietary therapy and pharmacologic therapy consistent with NCEP[41,42] and AHA/ACC[37] guidelines, educate and counsel on weight management, smoking cessation, and alcohol consumption as indicated, advise on increasing daily physical activity, increase dietary intake of plant stanol/sterols and viscous fiber **Expected outcomes:** Achieve and maintain lipids at targeted goals consistent with the AHA/ACC[37] recommendations
Diabetes management	**Evaluation:** Confirm diagnosis of diabetes based on established standards (American Diabetes Association [ADA][39] in United States, ESC[36] in Europe), obtain focused medical history related to potential complications (heart, vascular, vision, renal, distal extremity changes, autonomic and peripheral neuropathies), assess signs and symptoms associated with hypoglycemia/hyperglycemia, physical examination of potential sequelae, obtain fasting plasma glucose (FPG) and glycosylated hemoglobin (HbA1c) levels, identify patient's medication and diet regimens and assess effectiveness, assess patient blood sugar monitoring technique and compliance to monitoring **Interventions:** Educate patient on signs and symptoms of hypoglycemia/hyperglycemia, self-monitoring of blood glucose, exercise, injection sites (if appropriate), hydration, provide consultation with registered dietician for medical nutrition therapy, develop tailored individualized programs based on ADA recommendations[39] **Expected outcomes:** Communicate/coordinate with primary care physician or endocrinologist regarding signs and symptoms, medication control and adherence, compliance with self-monitoring of blood sugars, attain targeted FPG levels of 90–130 mg/dL and HbA1c <7%, minimal to no bouts of hypoglycemia/hyperglycemia

(continued on next page)

Table 4
(continued)

Core Components	Patient-Centered Medical Care and Management
Tobacco cessation	Evaluation: Verify smoking status and use of other tobacco products, obtain past smoking history and amount (if applicable), assess exposure to secondhand smoke (at home and work), determine patient readiness to quit smoking or using other tobacco products, evaluate psychosocial barriers to patient quitting Interventions: If patient is not ready to quit, provide motivational message based on the "5 Rs" (relevance, risks, rewards, roadblocks, and repetition),[43] if patient is ready to quit use the "5As" (ask, advise, assess, assist, and arrange)[44] to assist patient, consider recommending individualized or group counseling for smoking cessation, advise patient on arranging social support for cessation efforts, consult with physician regarding possible pharmacotherapy assistance, consider alternative therapies (acupuncture, hypnosis), educate and practice relapse-management skills with patient, follow-up with patient regularly Expected outcomes: A clearly delineated plan/strategy to achieve smoking cessation, adherence to program strategies and pharmacotherapy, patient knowledgeable in relapse prevention/management, long-term achievement to complete abstinence from smoking and other tobacco products
Psychosocial management	Evaluation: Assess for clinically significant levels of psychological distress (depression, anxiety, anger, hostility) and social distress (low socioeconomic status, isolation, marital/family problems, sexual dysfunction, substance abuse), identify psychotropic medications patient is prescribed and compliance with these medications, evaluate strategies for managing distress Interventions: Referral for counseling with professionals having expertise in managing psychosocial distress/conditions, possibly include significant others (family, partners) in counseling sessions, develop a supportive environment in the CR/secondary prevention program, educate in and support the use of self-help strategies by patients, in conjunction with primary care provider, consider use of pharmacotherapy, educate patient in monitoring for indicators of relapse Expected outcomes: Emotional well-being of patient, absence of clinically significant psychological and social distresses, patient adherence to medications, patient knowledgeable in relapse management/action plan

Physical activity counseling	Evaluation: Assess current physical activity level (home/work/recreational), compare activities to typical and relevant age/gender activity levels, assess readiness to increase activity if sedentary, self-efficacy and social support to make changes, and potential barriers to changing physical activity level Interventions: Provide education, counsel, and support for the benefits of physical activity, develop a plan in conjunction with the patient (as well as caregiver/family) to progressively increase physical activity 5–7 d/wk, individualize the progression of physical activity to minimize risk of musculoskeletal injury, continuous reassessment of plan with patient input, educate patient on relapse management Expected outcomes: Increased physical level of participation in home/work/recreational activities, improved psychosocial well-being, functional independence, prevention of disability, long-term adherence to maintaining physically active lifestyle, patient knowledgeable in relapse management/action plan
Exercise training	Evaluation: Symptom-limited exercise test (strongly recommended) before exercise-based CR program, thorough assessment of patient's physiologic responses (heart rate and rhythm, blood pressure, signs/symptoms, ST-segment changes, hemodynamics, perceived exertion, exercise capacity), determine risk stratification[33] of patient to decide on appropriate level of monitoring during exercise training Interventions: Develop/implement an individualized exercise prescription for patient based on evaluative findings and approved by the medical director or referring physician, exercise intervention should include aerobic, resistance, and flexibility training and address the prescriptive elements of frequency, intensity, duration, modalities, and progression,[34] advise/counsel patient on supplemental exercises and physical activities to incorporate into everyday lifestyle, educate on warning signs and symptoms to monitor during exercise Expected outcomes: Patient achieves improved cardiopulmonary fitness, strength, muscle endurance, and flexibility; reduced cardiovascular risk and risk of mortality; patient knowledgeable in self-monitoring warning signs

Table 5
Cardiac rehabilitation-recommendations and guidelines in heart failure

Reference		
Ades et al,[47] 2013	Considerations	• CR exercise training • HF self-care counseling
	Description of components	• Pretraining exercise testing (peak V_{O_2} and VE-V_{CO_2} slope); exercise prescription, volume (3–7 MET-h/wk); intensity 55%–80% heart rate reserve or 12–14 Borg perceived exertion; duration and frequency up-titrated before intensity increased; frequency 4 d/wk; duration >30 min/session; resistance training 2–3 times/wk major muscle groups using 1–2 sets of 10–12 repetitions/set • System for medications; limiting dietary sodium 2–2.3 g/d; avoid excess fluid intake <1.5–2 L/d; daily weights; signs and symptoms of worsening failure; provider contact if increased weight or increasing symptoms; smoking cessation; restrict alcohol intake and recreational drugs; treat depression and anxiety; assess for sleep disturbance; regular provider visits, monitor coexisting conditions such as high blood pressure, diabetes, and cholesterol abnormalities; maintain current immunizations (flu and pneumonia vaccine)
CMS,[45] 2014	Considerations	CR to beneficiaries with stable, chronic HF (left ventricular ejection fraction <35%, NYHA class II–IV symptoms despite being on optimal HF therapy for at least 6 wk. Stable patients defined as patients who have not had recent (<6 wk) or planned (<6 mo) major cardiovascular hospitalizations or procedures
	Description of components	• Essential elements of CR; physician supervision required • Physician-prescribed exercise in physician's office or hospital outpatient setting • Cardiac risk factor modification including education, counseling, and behavioral intervention • Psychosocial assessment • Outcomes assessment
Corra et al,[46] 2005	Considerations	• Clinical assessment • Identification and management of chronic HF-related disease • Pharmacologic approach • Nonpharmacologic approach; management of comorbidities • Exercise training • Psychological support
	Description of components	• History, physical, cardiac imaging, functional capacity, cardiac rhythm, fluid status • Depression, anemia, renal insufficiency, cachexia, atrial fibrillation, sleep disorders • Guideline-based therapy • Education and support for patient and caregiver • Individually tailored (depression, anxiety, social support)

Keteyian et al,[48] 2014	Considerations	• Assurance of clinical stability and optimal HF therapy • Patient assessment by CR staff for any "red flags," heart rate, blood pressure, and body weight at each visit • Assessment of functional/exercise capacity • Assessment of health-related quality of life • Dietary assessment with emphasis on sodium and fluid • Sleep apnea screening • Patient education and disease management
	Description of components	• No cardiovascular hospitalization (HF-related event) in the past 6 wk, optimization of HF therapy if new HF diagnosis and no planned cardiovascular hospitalization or procedure for the next 6 mo • Red flags: weight gain ≥3 lb since last visit or 5 lb in 1 wk, worsening dyspnea, excessive fatigue, swelling of legs or abdomen, productive cough, nocturia, orthopnea or paroxysmal nocturnal dyspnea, difficulty concentrating, implantable cardioverter defibrillator shock • Peak oxygen uptake from cardiopulmonary exercise test, 6-min walk test, or muscle strength (quadriceps 1-repetition maximum and handgrip strength) • Minnesota Living with HF, Kansas City Cardiomyopathy Questionnaire, Beck Depression Inventory, or Patient Health Questionnaire-9 • Registered dietician
Pina,[49] 2010	Considerations	• Exercise prescription • Patient education
	Description of components	• Type of exercise: aerobic, resistive, or both • Intensity (dose): 60%–70% peak HR (from complete physical examination), 70% HR reserve (consider β-blocker therapy), 13–14 Borg scale RPE, HR at ventilatory threshold or at 60%–80% maximum Vo_2 • Frequency: number of times/wk (most days per wk) • Duration: Per session, consider warm-up and cool-down, number of wk • Progression: low-level early, increase as tolerated • Dietary guidelines, risk factor modification, secondary prevention, education about HF and when to call for symptoms, smoking cessation counseling, and personal counseling if needed

(continued on next page)

Table 5
(continued)

		Reference
Wise,[50] 2007	Considerations	• Patient assessment • Nutritional counseling • Lipid management • Hypertension management • Smoking cessation • Diabetes management • Psychosocial management • Other education and counseling • Physical activity counseling • Exercise training
	Description of components	• History, physical, care plan development • Combined diet, exercise, and behavioral program • Nutritional counseling, weight management, exercise, alcohol moderation, and pharmacologic therapy • Lifestyle modifications (exercise, weight management, sodium restriction, alcohol moderation, smoking cessation, and pharmacologic therapy) • Support and appropriate treatment strategies • Dietary adherence and weight control (exercise, pharmacologic therapy, and risk factor control) • Individual or small-group education and counseling regarding HF, stress management, and health-related lifestyle change • Medications, investigations, and procedures, cardiac health beliefs and misconceptions, importance of follow-up by cardiology and primary care • Advice, support, and counseling. Assistance with return to work • Individualized exercise prescription for aerobic and resistance training based on risk stratification, patient and program goals, and resources; prescription should specify frequency, intensity, duration, and modalities; written guidelines to include home walking program

Adapted from Refs.[45–50]

Table 6
Patient, system, and provider level barriers to exercise in heart failure

Barriers to Exercise in HF	Balady et al,[55] 2011	Barbour & Miller,[56] 2008	Conraads et al,[57] 2012	Piepoli et al,[18] 2011	Tierney et al,[58] 2011	van der Wal et al,[59] 2006
Patient level						
Lack of motivation	—	●	●	●	●	—
Fear of overdoing	—	—	—	—	●	—
Lack of energy	—	—	—	—	—	●
Symptoms	—	—	●	●	●	●
Comorbid conditions	●	—	●	●	●	—
Lack of time (work and family obligations)	●	●	●	●	—	—
Older age	●	—	●	—	—	—
Financial concerns (low socioeconomic)	●	●	●	●	●	—
Depression	—	●	●	—	—	—
Lack of social support	●	●	—	●	●	—
Lower educational level	●	—	●	●	—	—
Inclement weather	—	—	—	—	●	—
Transportation issues	●	—	●	●	—	—
Duration and complexity of exercise	—	—	—	●	—	—
Attitude toward exercise	—	—	—	●	●	—
Minority status	●	—	●	—	—	—
Lack of insight into benefits of exercise	●	—	●	—	—	—
Level of disability	—	—	●	—	—	—
Overprotectiveness of family members	—	—	—	—	●	—
Cognitive problems	—	—	●	—	—	—
Lower self-efficacy	●	●	—	—	—	—
Low health literacy	●	—	—	—	—	—
System level						
Lack of referral	●	—	●	—	—	—
Lack of exercise sites/programs	●	—	●	●	●	—
Lack of resources and support	—	—	●	—	●	—
Lack of reimbursement	—	—	●	—	—	—
Provider level						
Providers cautioning against activity	—	—	—	—	●	—
Provider lack of belief in value of exercise	—	—	—	●	—	—
Lack of education about exercise benefits	—	—	●	—	—	—
Lack of educated personnel (HF expertise)	—	—	●	●	—	—
Strength of endorsement by physician	●	—	—	—	—	—

●, Specific barrier reported.
Adapted from Refs.[18,55–59]

personnel to direct and implement early inpatient CR. Addressing CR in inpatient settings is necessary to improve referrals and participation in outpatient CR. Arena and colleagues[62] discussed future directions that should include promoting a better understanding of outpatient CR as a cost-effective, multidisciplinary secondary prevention treatment option and chronic disease management service. Increasing referrals and participation of patients with HF in CR could be promoted by inclusion of HF chronic disease management in the delivery of CR. A HF disease management component is currently not specified in the guidelines, but it should be considered with an anticipated increase in the number of patients with HF being referred and participating in CR programs.

Inclusion of HF disease management as a core component in CR could be approached similarly to the way in which diabetes management has been included as a core component for CR. This approach would help to insure an appropriately tailored and individualized treatment plan for patients with HF participating in CR. Inclusion of HF disease management would have definite implications for the team and the core competencies of that team. Review of the position statement of Hamm and colleagues[63] from the AACVPR provides an excellent summary of core competencies for CR and secondary prevention professionals. This position statement did not include HF disease management in the list of core competencies. Hamm and colleagues[63] emphasized that one single health care professional cannot possess all the recommended core competencies. Rather, each member of the multidisciplinary team should contribute certain core competencies to the collective team based on education, training, and certifications or licensure. In an effective HF management program, Jaarsma[64] discussed the need to establish which health care provider will attend to each specific component of the overall plan. Essential to this process would be identification of the team leader, who would serve as the primary point person to coordinate the efforts of the team. Jaarsma[64] also emphasized the need to tailor a program to the individual patient situation because there is not a "one-size-fits-all" model. Finally, addition of a HF disease management component to CR would necessitate that providers with HF expertise be included as team members to assist in management of patients with HF participating in CR.

SUMMARY

The estimated cost of treating patients with HF in the United States is expected to more than double by 2030.[65] This forecast of the impact of HF in the United States should serve as a call to action. Despite well-documented benefits, participation in exercise training and CR programs by patients with HF remains low. In this article, standards and guidelines for exercise and CR in HF were reviewed. Although traditional CR had core components, it lacked care management specific for HF. Chronic stable HF patients can safely exercise; however, there are many unique needs that are not currently addressed at the patient, system, and provider levels. As we face economic and political forces that are expected to require major change to the health care delivery system, it becomes even more important to capitalize on the advantages that come with team-based care. CR has always served as a model of team-based care; however, the model must now include professionals with HF expertise to guide patients in safe exercise and self-management strategies appropriate for this chronically ill population.

REFERENCES

1. O'Connor CM, Whellan DJ, Lee KL, et al. Efficacy and safety of exercise training in patients with chronic heart failure: HF-ACTION randomized controlled trial. JAMA 2009;301(14):1439–50.
2. Taylor RS, Piepoli MF, Smart N, et al. Exercise training for chronic heart failure (ExTraMATCH II): protocol for an individual participant data meta-analysis. Int J Cardiol 2014;174(3):683–7.
3. Alves AJ, Ribeiro F, Goldhammer E, et al. Exercise training improves diastolic function in heart failure patients. Med Sci Sports Exerc 2012;44(5):776–85.
4. Edelmann F, Gelbrich G, Düngen H, et al. Exercise training improves exercise capacity and diastolic function in patients with heart failure with preserved ejection fraction: results of the ex-DHF (Exercise training in Diastolic Heart Failure) pilot study. J Am Coll Cardiol 2011;58(17):1780–91.
5. Haykowsky MJ, Brubaker PH, Stewart KP, et al. Effect of endurance training on the determinants of peak exercise oxygen consumption in elderly patients with stable compensated heart failure and preserved ejection fraction. J Am Coll Cardiol 2012;60(2):120–8.
6. Kitzman DW, Brubaker PH, Morgan TM, et al. Exercise training in older patients with heart failure and preserved ejection fraction: a randomized, controlled, single-blind trial. Circ Heart Fail 2010; 3(6):659–67.
7. Kitzman DW, Brubaker PH, Herrington DM, et al. Effect of endurance exercise training on endothelial function and arterial stiffness in older patients with heart failure and preserved ejection fraction: a

randomized, controlled, single-blind trial. J Am Coll Cardiol 2013;62(7):584–92.

8. Smart NA, Haluska B, Jeffriess L, et al. Exercise training in heart failure with preserved systolic function: a randomized controlled trial of the effects on cardiac function and functional capacity. Congest Heart Fail 2012;18(6):295–301.

9. Taylor RS, Davies EJ, Dalal HM, et al. Effects of exercise training for heart failure with preserved ejection fraction: a systematic review and meta-analysis of comparative studies. Int J Cardiol 2012; 162(1):6–13.

10. Thirapatarapong W, Thomas RJ, Pack Q, et al. Commercial insurance coverage for outpatient cardiac rehabilitation in patients with heart failure in the United States. J Cardiopulm Rehabil Prev 2014; 34(6):386–9.

11. Yancy CW, Jessup M, Bozkurt B, et al. 2013 ACCF/AHA guideline for the management of heart failure: a report of the American College of Cardiology Foundation/American Heart Association Task Force on Practice Guidelines. J Am Coll Cardiol 2013; 62(16):e147–239.

12. Lainscak M, Blue L, Clark AL, et al. Self-care management of heart failure: practical recommendations from the Patient Care Committee of the Heart Failure Association of the European Society of Cardiology. Eur J Heart Fail 2011;13(2):115–26.

13. Lindenfeld J, Albert NM, Boehmer JP, et al. Heart Failure Society of America (HFSA) 2010 comprehensive heart failure practice guideline. J Card Fail 2010;16(6):e1–194.

14. McMurray JJ, Adamopoulos S, Anker SD, et al. ESC guidelines for the diagnosis and treatment of acute and chronic heart failure 2012: the Task Force for the Diagnosis and Treatment of Acute and Chronic Heart Failure 2012 of the European Society of Cardiology. Developed in collaboration with the Heart Failure Association (HFA) of the ESC. Eur Heart J 2012; 33(14):1787–847.

15. National Institute for Health and Care Excellence. NICE quality standards [QS9]. 2011. Available at: https://www.nice.org.uk/guidance/qs9. Accessed December, 2014.

16. American Association of Cardiovascular and Pulmonary Rehabilitation. About cardiovascular & pulmonary rehabilitation. 2014. Available at: https://www.aacvpr.org/about/aboutcardiacpulmonaryrehab/tabid/560/default.aspx. Accessed December, 2014.

17. Adsett J, Mullins R. Evidence based guidelines for exercise and chronic heart failure. 2010. Available at: http://www.health.qld.gov.au/heart_failure/pdf/guide_exercise_chf.pdf. Accessed December, 2014.

18. Piepoli MF, Conraads V, Corra U, et al. Exercise training in heart failure: from theory to practice. A consensus document of the Heart Failure Association and the European Association for Cardiovascular Prevention and Rehabilitation. Eur J Heart Fail 2011;13(4):347–57.

19. Pina IL, Apstein CS, Balady GJ, et al. Exercise and heart failure: a statement from the American Heart Association committee on exercise, rehabilitation, and prevention. Circulation 2003;107(8):1210–25.

20. Selig SE, Levinger I, Williams AD, et al. Exercise & Sports Science Australia Position Statement on exercise training and chronic heart failure. J Sci Med Sport 2010;13(3):288–94.

21. Bartlo P. Evidence-based application of aerobic and resistance training in patients with congestive heart failure. J Cardiopulm Rehabil Prev 2007;27(6):368–75.

22. Braith RW, Beck DT. Resistance exercise: training adaptations and developing a safe exercise prescription. Heart Fail Rev 2008;13(1):69–79.

23. De Maeyer C, Beckers P, Vrints CJ, et al. Exercise training in chronic heart failure. Ther Adv Chronic Dis 2013;4(3):105–17.

24. Norman JF. ExPAAC proceedings: exercise training for individuals with heart failure. J Geriatr Phys Ther 2012;35(4):165–72.

25. Smart N, Fang ZY, Marwick TH. A practical guide to exercise training for heart failure patients. J Card Fail 2003;9(1):49–58.

26. Myers J. Principles of exercise prescription for patients with chronic heart failure. Heart Fail Rev 2008;13(1):61–8.

27. Davies EJ, Moxham T, Rees K, et al. Exercise based rehabilitation for heart failure. Cochrane Database Syst Rev 2010;(4):CD003331.

28. Downing J, Balady GJ. The role of exercise training in heart failure. J Am Coll Cardiol 2011;58(6):561–9.

29. Haykowsky MJ, Liang Y, Pechter D, et al. A meta-analysis of the effect of exercise training on left ventricular remodeling in heart failure patients: the benefit depends on the type of training performed. J Am Coll Cardiol 2007;49(24):2329–36.

30. Smart N. Exercise training for heart failure patients with and without systolic dysfunction: an evidence-based analysis of how patients benefit. Cardiol Res Pract 2010;2011:837238.

31. Smart N, Marwick TH. Exercise training for patients with heart failure: a systematic review of factors that improve mortality and morbidity. Am J Med 2004;116(10):693–706.

32. Tai MK, Meininger JC, Frazier LQ. A systematic review of exercise interventions in patients with heart failure. Biol Res Nurs 2008;10(2):156–82.

33. American Association of Cardiovascular and Pulmonary Rehabilitation. Guidelines for cardiac rehabilitation and secondary prevention programs. 5th edition. Champaign (IL): Human Kinetics Publishers; 2013.

34. Balady GJ, Williams MA, Ades PA, et al. Core components of cardiac rehabilitation/secondary prevention programs: 2007 update: a scientific statement from the American Heart Association exercise,

Cardiac Rehabilitation, and Prevention Committee, the Council on Clinical Cardiology; the Councils on Cardiovascular Nursing, Epidemiology and Prevention, and Nutrition, Physical Activity, and Metabolism; and the American Association of Cardiovascular and Pulmonary Rehabilitation. Circulation 2007;115(20):2675–82.

35. British Association for Cardiovascular Prevention and Rehabilitation. The BACPR standards and core components for cardiovascular disease prevention and rehabilitation 2012. London: British Cardiovascular Society; 2012.

36. Graham I, Atar D, Borch-Johnsen K, et al. European guidelines on cardiovascular disease prevention in clinical practice: full text. Fourth Joint Task Force of the European Society of Cardiology and other societies on cardiovascular disease prevention in clinical practice (constituted by representatives of nine societies and by invited experts). Eur J Cardiovasc Prev Rehabil 2007;14(Suppl 2):S1–113.

37. Smith SC Jr, Allen J, Blair SN, et al. AHA/ACC guidelines for secondary prevention for patients with coronary and other atherosclerotic vascular disease: 2006 update: endorsed by the National Heart, Lung, and Blood Institute. Circulation 2006; 113(19):2363–72.

38. Leon AS, Franklin BA, Costa F, et al. Cardiac rehabilitation and secondary prevention of coronary heart disease: an American Heart Association Scientific Statement from the Council on Clinical Cardiology (subcommittee on exercise, cardiac rehabilitation, and prevention) and the Council on Nutrition, Physical Activity, and Metabolism (subcommittee on physical activity), in collaboration with the American Association of Cardiovascular and Pulmonary Rehabilitation. Circulation 2005;111(3):369–76.

39. American Diabetes Association. Standards of medical care in diabetes–2014. Diabetes Care 2014; 37(Suppl 1):S14–80.

40. Chobanian AV, Bakris GL, Black HR, et al. The seventh report of the Joint National Committee on Prevention, Detection, Evaluation, and Treatment of High Blood Pressure: the JNC 7 report. JAMA 2003;289(19):2560–72.

41. National Cholesterol Education Program (NCEP) Expert Panel on Detection, Evaluation, and Treatment of High Blood Cholesterol in Adults (Adult Treatment Panel III). Third Report of the National Cholesterol Education Program (NCEP) Expert Panel on Detection, Evaluation, and Treatment of High Blood Cholesterol in Adults (Adult Treatment Panel III) Final Report. Circulation 2002;106(25): 3143–421.

42. Grundy SM, Cleeman JI, Merz CN, et al. Implications of recent clinical trials for the national cholesterol education program adult treatment panel III guidelines. Circulation 2004;110(2):227–39.

43. Agency for Healthcare Research and Quality. Patients not ready to make a quit attempt now (the "5 R's"). 2012. Available at: http://www.ahrq.gov/professionals/clinicians-providers/guidelines-recommendations/tobacco/5rs.html. Accessed December, 2014.

44. Agency for Healthcare Research and Quality. Five major steps to intervention (the "5 A's"). 2012. Available at: http://www.ahrq.gov/professionals/clinicians-providers/guidelines-recommendations/tobacco/5steps.html. Accessed December, 2014.

45. Centers for Medicare & Medicaid Services. Decision memo for cardiac rehabilitation (CR) programs - chronic heart failure. 2014. Available at: http://www.cms.gov/medicare-coverage-database/details/nca-decision-memo.aspx?NCAId=270. Accessed December, 2014.

46. Corra U, Giannuzzi P, Adamopoulos S, et al. Executive summary of the position paper of the Working Group on Cardiac Rehabilitation and Exercise Physiology of the European Society of Cardiology (ESC): core components of cardiac rehabilitation in chronic heart failure. Eur J Cardiovasc Prev Rehabil 2005; 12(4):321–5.

47. Ades PA, Keteyian SJ, Balady GJ, et al. Cardiac rehabilitation exercise and self-care for chronic heart failure. JACC Heart Fail 2013;1(6):540–7.

48. Keteyian SJ, Squires RW, Ades PA, et al. Incorporating patients with chronic heart failure into outpatient cardiac rehabilitation: practical recommendations for exercise and self-care counseling—a clinical review. J Cardiopulm Rehabil Prev 2014;34(4):223–32.

49. Pina IL. Cardiac rehabilitation in heart failure: a brief review and recommendations. Curr Cardiol Rep 2010;12(3):223–9.

50. Wise FM. Exercise based cardiac rehabilitation in chronic heart failure. Aust Fam Physician 2007; 36(12):1019–24.

51. Pack QR, Squires RW, Lopez-Jimenez F, et al. The current and potential capacity for cardiac rehabilitation utilization in the United States. J Cardiopulm Rehabil Prev 2014;34(5):318–26.

52. Bethell HJ, Evans JA, Turner SC, et al. The rise and fall of cardiac rehabilitation in the United Kingdom since 1998. J Public Health (Oxf) 2007;29(1):57–61.

53. Bjarnason-Wehrens B, McGee H, Zwisler AD, et al. Cardiac rehabilitation in Europe: results from the European Cardiac Rehabilitation Inventory Survey. Eur J Cardiovasc Prev Rehabil 2010;17(4):410–8.

54. Thomas RJ, King M, Lui K, et al. AACVPR/ACC/AHA 2007 performance measures on cardiac rehabilitation for referral to and delivery of cardiac rehabilitation/secondary prevention services. J Cardiopulm Rehabil Prev 2007;27(5):260–90.

55. Balady GJ, Ades PA, Bittner VA, et al. Referral, enrollment, and delivery of cardiac rehabilitation/secondary

prevention programs at clinical centers and beyond: a presidential advisory from the American Heart Association. Circulation 2011;124(25):2951–60.

56. Barbour KA, Miller NH. Adherence to exercise training in heart failure: a review. Heart Fail Rev 2008;13(1):81–9.

57. Conraads VM, Deaton C, Piotrowicz E, et al. Adherence of heart failure patients to exercise: barriers and possible solutions: a position statement of the Study Group on Exercise Training in Heart Failure of the Heart Failure Association of the European Society of Cardiology. Eur J Heart Fail 2012;14(5):451–8.

58. Tierney S, Elwers H, Sange C, et al. What influences physical activity in people with heart failure? A qualitative study. Int J Nurs Stud 2011;48(10):1234–43.

59. van der Wal MH, Jaarsma T, Moser DK, et al. Compliance in heart failure patients: the importance of knowledge and beliefs. Eur Heart J 2006;27(4):434–40.

60. Brown TM, Hernandez AF, Bittner V, et al. Predictors of cardiac rehabilitation referral in coronary artery disease patients: findings from the American Heart Association's Get with the Guidelines Program. J Am Coll Cardiol 2009;54(6):515–21.

61. King M, Bittner V, Josephson R, et al. Medical director responsibilities for outpatient cardiac rehabilitation/secondary prevention programs: 2012 update: a statement for health care professionals from the American Association of Cardiovascular and Pulmonary Rehabilitation and the American Heart Association. Circulation 2012; 126(21):2535–43.

62. Arena R, Williams M, Forman DE, et al. Increasing referral and participation rates to outpatient cardiac rehabilitation: the valuable role of healthcare professionals in the inpatient and home health settings: a science advisory from the American Heart Association. Circulation 2012;125(10):1321–9.

63. Hamm LF, Sanderson BK, Ades PA, et al. Core competencies for cardiac rehabilitation/secondary prevention professionals: 2010 update: position statement of the American Association of Cardiovascular and Pulmonary Rehabilitation. J Cardiopulm Rehabil Prev 2011;31(1):2–10.

64. Jaarsma T. Health care professionals in a heart failure team. Eur J Heart Fail 2005;7(3):343–9.

65. Heidenreich PA, Albert NM, Allen LA, et al. Forecasting the impact of heart failure in the United States: a policy statement from the American Heart Association. Circ Heart Fail 2013;6(3):606–19.

Team-Based Care for External Telemonitoring in Patients with Heart Failure

Josie Dimengo, MSN, RN[a],*, Gerrye Stegall, MN, RN[b]

KEYWORDS

- Heart failure • Telemonitoring • Remote monitoring • Disease management • mHealth
- HF*/therapy • Telemetry/*methods • Behavior change

KEY POINTS

- Heart failure telemonitoring studies to date are inconclusive and not generalizable.
- Addition of proven strategies, such as behavior change theory and disease management programs, to telemonitoring may increase effectiveness.
- Increased availability and popularity of wearable monitoring devices may increase adherence to telemonitoring, and decrease costs of care.

INTRODUCTION

Healthy people cost less and are more productive. This may seem an odd perspective when discussing patients with heart failure (HF). Multiple studies have been conducted assessing strategies for managing HF with the goal of decreasing admissions and readmissions, decreasing mortality, and ultimately increasing self-management and improving quality of life (QOL). There is no silver bullet in managing these complex patients, who have a condition that is progressive and incurable. From the plethora of clinical trials, it is well established that optimal medication management contributes to a decrease in hospital readmissions and mortality.[1] Telemonitoring has been explored as an intervention to support and monitor adherence to all aspects of the HF management plan, including medication and appointment adherence, diet, exercise, and self-care. Initial studies comparing usual care with telemonitoring interventions looked promising, reporting a decrease in hospital admissions and mortality.[2–5] However, two large-scale randomized trials comparing telemonitoring with structured telephonic support showed no statistically significant differences in outcomes.[6] This article addresses the findings of these studies and provides recommendations for future consideration. The need to apply the right interventions, to the right patient, at the right time, based on self-efficacy and readiness to change, is also addressed. Ultimately, involving patients in decision-making increases the likelihood of adherence to recommended interventions and maintenance of health and productivity.

WHY USE TELEMONITORING?

Although disease progression impacts readmissions, one-half to two-thirds of hospital readmissions are avoidable.[7] Providing interventions that add clarity to a patient's prescribed HF action plan, insight into the consequences of nonadherence, and assessing not only the patient's readiness to change, but also their confidence in doing so, may contribute to optimal HF

Disclosure Statement: No disclosures.
[a] Healthways, Inc., Employer Market, 701 Cool Springs Boulevard, Franklin, TN 37067, USA; [b] Healthways International, 701 Cool Springs Boulevard, Franklin, TN 37067, USA
* Corresponding author.
E-mail address: josie.dimengo@healthways.com

Heart Failure Clin 11 (2015) 451–465
http://dx.doi.org/10.1016/j.hfc.2015.03.008
1551-7136/15/$ – see front matter Published by Elsevier Inc.

heartfailure.theclinics.com

management.[8,9] Thus, the question becomes, how do we best support patients with chronic HF in the outpatient setting? Which strategies can we leverage to ultimately keep patients in their healthiest state possible, allowing them to be productive? How can technology be used to support the behavior change that is needed for them to adopt and maintain healthier lifestyle habits? Finally, what systems can be put into place to incorporate timely outpatient patient measurement data into the hospital record to help decrease preventable (and nonreimbursed) readmissions?

Telemonitoring has been proposed as a potential solution to more closely monitor daily activities, and to facilitate awareness and education on the cause and effect of daily life choices, specifically related to diet and symptom management. The goals of telemonitoring include early detection of clinical deterioration; increasing outpatient management "touchpoints" that are cost-effective; empowering patients to self-manage HF, leading to adoption of a healthier lifestyle and avoiding frequent exacerbations; improving coordination of care across multiple disciplines, inpatient and outpatient[3]; and collaborative decision-making among patients, family members/significant others, and providers.[1,2,7,10] Outcome measurements include mortality (all-cause and/or cardiovascular), number of emergency department visits, HF readmissions, QOL, self-care management, and patients' acceptance of the intervention.[11–13]

First-generation telemonitoring systems provided patients with a blood pressure cuff to monitor pulse and blood pressure, a scale to monitor weight, and a hub that used a landline telephone to transmit the information to a central repository. Health care providers, typically nurses, would monitor and respond to readings that fell outside established parameters.[2,5,13,14] The rapid growth of technology, such as Bluetooth and videoconferencing, has dramatically increased capabilities for data acquisition and transmission, and the capability to use additional clinical assessment tools, such as electrocardiogram and pulse oximetry.[9] **Table 1** provides an overview of capabilities and factors that need to be considered when developing telemonitoring initiatives.

Fig. 1 is an overview of the interventions provided to a patient with HF from time of identification to time of deinstallation of telemonitoring with nonmobile devices.

DOES TELEMONITORING WORK?

Multiple studies were completed to assess the additive value of telemonitoring to usual HF care.

Varying sample sizes and patient characteristics (age, ethnicity, New York Heart Association [NYHA] class, length of study interventions provided) made comparative analysis of the studies difficult. Interpretation of findings was complex because of poorly defined terminology, such as "usual care" or disease management (DM) versus case management, types of interventions provided (video-conferencing, structured telephonic calls, interactive voice recognition), alternate methods of data transmission and data points captured, invasive monitoring for patients with implantable devices, and measurement of different end points. Additional services, such as management in outpatient HF clinics, home health care visits, interventions provided by nurses practicing within physician offices versus those delivered through vendor call centers providing the technology, or DM program interventions further complicated the comparison of impact on outcomes. For example, intervention variations included an ability to adjust medication regimens or provide additional HF education when a triggering alert occurred, adding a human element, whereas other systems used a technology-triggered intervention when alerts were generated. To assist in categorizing and collating study outcomes, several systematic reviews and meta-analyses were conducted, with some including only studies with robust study designs, adequate sample sizes, and telemonitoring provided in community setting.[11–15] An overview of these studies that included only noninvasive telemonitoring interventions is provided in **Table 2**.

Although there were individual beneficial end points noted in several trials, findings were not consistent. When study authors compared telemonitoring with usual care, researchers found a decrease in hospital admissions and mortality.[3–5,11] Although increases in QOL were reported, they were not statistically significant.[2,14,16,17] Overall, telemonitoring using either telephonic nurse support or automated telemonitoring reduced hospital admissions and all-cause mortality by nearly one-fifth.[1]

However, in studies where direct comparison of telemonitoring with telephonic nurse support was examined, no difference in outcomes was noted.[6] The variations in study characteristics make it difficult to establish generalizable conclusions about the effectiveness of telemonitoring. Other findings suggest that telemonitoring added cost and complexity to the care of patients with HF without adding benefit over self-monitoring with telephonic nurse support.[3] Few studies explain how data collected support clinical decision-making and interventions.[18]

Table 1
Telemonitoring considerations: patient selection, intervention type, and operational processes

Physiologic factors available for HF telemonitoring	Heart rate (obtained via automated BP cuff) BP (obtained via automated BP cuff) Weight (obtained via digital scales) ECG (obtained via transmittable ECG mobile unit technology) Oxygen saturation (obtained via automated pulse oximetry) Peak flow Heart and/or lung sounds (obtained via Bluetooth-enabled technology) Activity level using pedometers or mobile phone sensors
Types of interventions	Text or telephone call reminders to complete daily measurements IVR technology (one- or two-way) System-generated symptom questions when readings are out of range Quizzes to assess HF self-care knowledge HF education Individualized messaging to patients Videoconferencing/assessment capability Reporting/printouts for patient to share with physicians during visits (sent electronically or patient to print)

Patient considerations	Selection criteria
	In-home space limitations for telemonitoring equipment
	Patient's ability to use the equipment:
	    Ability to assemble the equipment
	    Stability to stand on the scale: standard scale vs stand up scale with handlebars
	    Dexterity to use the BP cuff, mobile phone, or other monitoring collaterals
	Selection of scales with upper weight limits that can be used for obese patients
	Increased number of alerts because of others in the household using the equipment
	Font size of telemonitoring screen displays and reading levels of applications used for patients to self-report symptoms
	Dexterity to use self-reporting applications
	TTY for the hearing impaired if IVR is a channel used for telephonic intervention
	Portability of equipment to ensure daily adherence particularly during extended periods away from home
	Carrier fees associated with texting on mobile devices
	Multilingual capabilities

Operational considerations	Cost considerations
	    Telemonitoring equipment (who pays, short- and long-term)
	    Staff needed to monitor alerts and provide telephonic outreach support (RN vs MD)
	    Technology and licensure needed to ensure secure transfer of patient-specific data that support HIPAA compliance
	    Method of alert monitoring and cost associated if centralized data repository is used
	    Integration of patient information into the electronic health record
	Other
	    Development of clinical parameters that require intervention; upper and lower limits of heart rate/BP measurement; weight, daily and weekly increases; acceptability of individualizing these to each patient as needed vs using standard settings
	    Establishing standard guidelines/processes for alert monitoring of physiologic data and IVR responses requiring action
	    Number of alerts allowed to exceed the limits before clinician action is generated
	    Duration of telemonitoring and replacement once patient is proficient at self-monitoring
	    Clear expectations on accountability for responding to alerts
	    Graduation criteria used to identify when telemonitoring devices can be removed and process to retrieve equipment
	    Storage of consent forms
	    Legal issues associated with nonresponse to urgent/emergent alerts
	    Physician/health system reimbursement for telemonitoring services

(continued on next page)

Table 1
(continued)

Outcome measurement	Outcomes typically measured HF-specific vs all-cause hospital admissions/readmissions ED visits Inpatient length of stay All-cause mortality Changes in patterns of use (decrease ED or HDC, but increase in outpatient visits) Effect on overall health outcomes Health-related QOL, perception of health Patient satisfaction with interventions Health care cost savings for HF patients Cost/benefit analysis Return on investment

Abbreviations: BP, blood pressure; ECG, electrocardiogram; ED, emergency department; HDC, hospital discharge; HF, heart failure; HIPAA, Health Insurance Portability and Accountability Act; IVR, interactive voice response; MD, medical doctor; QOL, quality of life; RN, registered nurse; TTY, teletypewriter technology.
Adapted from Refs.[2,9–11,13,18,19,22,23]

Additional outcomes were gleaned from select studies. Telemonitoring was not advantageous for patients with advanced HF.[14,16] This may not be directly related to the intervention itself or lack of focus on self-care, but rather to the natural progression of the disease process. The benefits of telemonitoring were greater in longer-term studies than those following patients for shorter time frames.[11] Compliance was generally reported to be high, ranging from 75% to 99%.[12] Older patients (age 70 years or greater) benefited from both telemonitoring programs and did not require more resources to support the intervention.[11,19]

Patient and practitioner perceptions of telemonitoring services also varied.[20,21] Patients found it useful and reassuring that someone was paying attention to their clinical status, leading to a decrease in anxiety. Patients felt more aware of their HF condition and more empowered. They liked surveillance during the study, but voiced concern that continuing long-term "surveillance" impacted their freedom (eg, they did not like "big brother" constantly watching them). Alternatively, many patients were willing to partially fund telemonitoring for ongoing use.[21] Practitioners found telemonitoring useful and believed that it allowed patients to better manage themselves with access to ongoing physiologic data.[20] Practitioners believed red flag alerts provided an ability to leverage "teachable" moments in guiding patients to self-management, but were concerned about growing dependence on the device (reactive), rather than on self-management (proactive).[20] Finally, practitioners were concerned about an increase in their workload and ongoing costs of providing telemonitoring.[20]

Perception of improvement in health status was reported by patients surveyed 3 months following removal of telemonitoring equipment.[22] Self-care improved, because 97% of patients reported the program assisted them to take better care of themselves. All noted they had an HF action plan and 81% made positive dietary changes.[22]

Ultimately, the benefit of telemonitoring is inconclusive. Additional studies need to be conducted that focus on multidisciplinary interventions that can reduce rates of HF hospitalization, with consideration to specific patient characteristics that may be important predictors of HF and other cardiac disease–related survival and hospitalization.[1,7,18]

TELEMONITORING COSTS

Providing telemonitoring services comes with cost implications that have not been well-established, but must be considered before implementation. Patient-incurred equipment costs, particularly if cellular technology is used (equipment and monthly cellular phone/data charges), and capital expenditure for a centralized monitoring system or integration into an electronic health record must be evaluated. The cost of staff needed to monitor and respond to daily alerts, along with additional minutes for troubleshooting, intervention, or patient education, must be included in assessing overall operational expenses. A comprehensive overview of inpatient and outpatient costs including pharmacy, telephonic, and face-to-face contacts with generalists and specialists and other services (home health care, sessions with psychologists and physiotherapists) should be considered when assessing cost-effectiveness of telemonitoring.[23]

Very few studies have been completed that address the cost of noninvasive telemonitoring

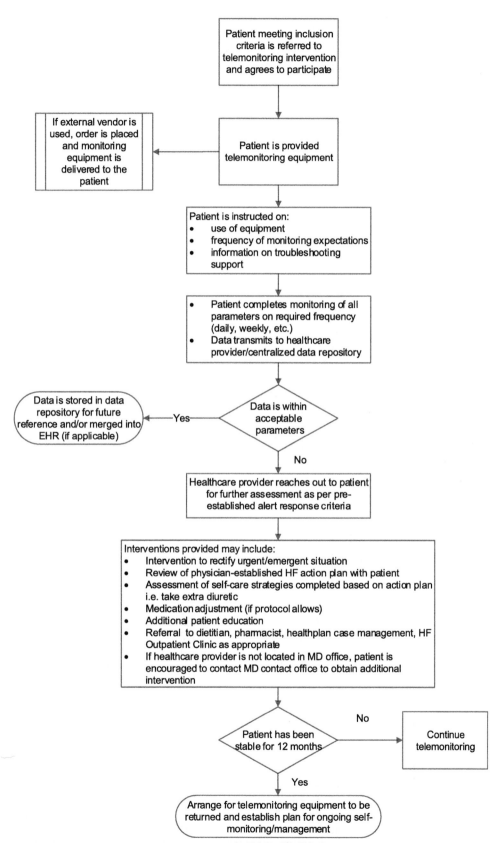

Fig. 1. Overview of the telemonitoring process. EHR, electronic health record.

Table 2
Overview of heart failure telemonitoring randomized control trials comparing usual care versus telemonitoring interventions

Reference, Study Date	Study Group Interventions	Study Duration (Months)	Sample Size	Outcomes: Positive	Outcomes: Neutral (No Effect)	Comments
Usual Care vs Telemonitoring Interventions						
Goldberg et al,[16] 2003 WHARF Trial	Daily transmission of weight and symptom reporting using telemonitoring device	6	280	↓Mortality (all cause) = 56.2% ↑QOL: NSS	HOSP - HF (no difference) LOS EDVs	NYHA III and IV Primary end point of 6-mo rehospitalization, no difference from UC Optimal/aggressive medication management 98.5% compliance with monitoring reported
Weintraub et al,[2] 2010 SPAN-CHF II	HF DM + automated HM system	3	188	↓Mortality ↓HOSP (HF) ↓LOS	EDVs HOSP (all-cause) QOL	NYHA II and III An estimated 15%–20% increase in DM intervention caused by telemonitoring
Chaudhry et al,[41] 2010 Tele-HF study	Patients required to call into IVR system to report daily weight and respond to questions related to HF symptoms	6	1653	None	HOSP (all-cause) HOSP (HF) LOS Mortality	Participation decreased to 55% at 26 wk with reporting only 3 d per week
Koehler et al,[42] 2011 TIM-HF	Daily transmission of ECG, BP, and weight via cell phone	26	710	None	Mortality (all-cause) HOSP (all-cause) (NSS) LOS EDVs QOL	NYHA II and III Intervention provided by physicians 81% participation with 70% providing daily data

Study	Intervention	Duration (mo)	N	Outcomes improved	Outcomes no impact	Other
Dendale et al,[3] 2012 TEMA-HF	Standard education course on HF and instruction on how to use electronic equipment and cell phone that transmitted weight, HR, and BP readings to PCP and OPD HF clinic: automated email alerts addressed	6	160	↓Mortality (all-cause) HF readmission rates ↓LOS	Readmission rates	NYHA class >II Increased costs in TM group
Boyne et al,[23] 2013 TEHAF-study	HF education, two prescheduled HF clinic visits and telemonitoring device sending responses to preset questions addressing symptoms, HF knowledge and behavior. VS were not measured. Patients categorized as high risk received immediate RN intervention	12	382	↓HF readmission rates	Mortality HOSP (HF) for initial HOSP (no impact)	—
Baker et al,[4] 2011	Automated telemonitoring system	24	1767	↓Mortality (15% reduction) ↓HOSP (all-cause) 18% measured quarterly	LOS EDVs	HF and COPD Medicare beneficiaries

(continued on next page)

Table 2
(continued)

Reference, Study Date	Study Group Interventions	Study Duration (Months)	Sample Size	Outcomes: Positive	Outcomes: Neutral (No Effect)	Comments
Studies Comparing Usual Care vs Telemonitoring using Videoconferencing						
Woodend et al,[5] 2008	3 mo of weekly videoconferencing with RN to provide patient assessment and self-care education + daily transmission of BP/weight + occasional 12-lead ECG	12	249	↓HOSP (51% at 3 mo and 45% at 1 y) ↓LOS (21% reduction at 1 y)	EDV	NYHA II to IV Decreases in EDV and OPD cardiology visits between intervention and UC groups NSS at 1 y
Takahashi et al,[14] 2012	Daily symptom assessment and biometric readings transmitted to central station with RN outreach for alerts generated	12	205	None	↑Mortality (causes unknown) HOSP LOS EDV QOL	Older (mean age = 80), sicker patients with multiple comorbidities
Usual Care vs Telephonic Nurse Support vs Telemonitoring						
Cleland et al,[6] 2005 TEN-HMS	TM group: twice daily of BP, pulse, ECG, and weight measurement with automated telephone line transmission to central repository in hospital or clinic TNS group: monthly RN telephone calls without TM	8	426	↓Mortality in TNS (17%) and TM (29%, but NSS trend) ↓LOS for HF HOSP (6 d in TM group only)	↑ EDV in both intervention groups No difference in HOSP (all-cause) in two TM or TNS groups ↑mortality in UC group (45%)	NYHA II to IV Primary end point (reduction in days spent alive and out of hospital) = no statistical difference between TNS and TM Patient satisfaction with equipment = 96% Ease of use = 97%

| Mortara et al,[43] 2009 Struct Tele HHH Study | 12 | 461 | Weight, HR, BP, doses of medications taken, dyspnea, blood results three intervention groups: Group 1. TNS: monthly supportive telephone contacts to assess clinical status Group 2. TNS + TM with weekly transmission of vital signs/weight, BP, and symptoms and monthly 24-h cardiorespiratory recordings, which were not made available to the clinical team Group 3: Group 2 strategies + monthly 24-h recording of cardiorespiratory activity | ↓HOSP (all-cause) ↓Mortality (all-cause) | ↓LOS (NSS) ↓HOSP (HF) (NSS) | NYHA II - IV Adherence, 81% completion of vital signs; 92% completion of cardiorespiratory reading |

Abbreviations: BP, blood pressure; COPD, chronic obstructive pulmonary disease; DM, disease management; ECG, electrocardiogram; EDV, emergency department visits; HF, heart failure; HM, home monitoring; HOSP, hospitalizations; HR, heart rate; IVR, interactive voice recognition system; LOS, length of stay; NSS, not statistically significant; NYHA, New York Heart Association; OPD, outpatient visits; QOL, quality of life; RN, registered nurse; TM, telemonitoring; TNS, telephonic nurse support; UC, usual care; VS, vital signs.
Data from Refs.[2–6,11,13,14,23,41]

services provided to patients with HF in the community. Overall, no significant differences in mean overall costs were noted when comparing the usual care with telemonitoring study groups.[13,23,24] In a retrospective claims review of costs associated with a telemonitoring intervention, coupled with an HF DM program, researchers found a significant reduction in per member per month costs during the intervention time period (8–12 months) and in the postintervention period (6 months) after monitoring equipment was removed,[22] and outcomes were associated with decreased health care use (emergency department visits and hospital admissions/readmissions).

Payment for long-term use must be considered. In a qualitative study, 14 of 22 patients (64%) reported a willingness to pay for the technology.[21] Some patients suggested that having to pay a nominal fee might increase adherence to obtaining measurements. Others patients, however, noted they would not have the financial means to pay for technology and believed this should be considered a medical expense that insurance companies should pay for, or that employers should fund as part of their work benefits.[21]

TELEHEALTH REIMBURSEMENT

The Centers for Medicare and Medicare Services (CMS) supports grants designed to expand the use of technologies that promote better patient transitions from hospitals, rehabilitation centers, or nursing facilities back to homes or other community settings.[25] Use of such funds could support additional telemonitoring research.

CMS provides reimbursement for telemedicine services; however, patient eligibility guidelines and billing guidelines must be followed.[26–28] Effective in 2015, CMS added a procedural code for physician reimbursement for remote patient monitoring of chronic conditions.[29] Historically, Medicare did not pay separately for such services, requiring that billing be bundled with an "evaluation and management" code. Additional support for telemonitoring services may be available under state-specific Medicaid provisions or private payor as enacted by the Legislated Mandate for Private Coverage.[30]

LEVERAGING SELF-EFFICACY AND BEHAVIOR CHANGE STRATEGIES WITH TECHNOLOGY

Early detection of decompensation is one of the central goals of telemonitoring. Patient adherence to prescribed HF therapies is not optimal.[1,8] Behavior change concepts are often used to apply stage-matched interventions; however, patients'

motivation and confidence in initiating and sustaining self-care behaviors should also be considered.[8,31] Patients' perceptions of their stage of change may not always match their daily self-care behaviors.[31] Health behavior change is complex and requires the ability to tailor interventions that are right for each individual, and at the right time for the person to move them from considering benefits the change will provide to making and sustaining that change.[32] Sustained change is not achieved in patients who are not ready to change, because they have not internalized the need for change.[7] They may not know what change is required, do not see the importance or need to change, or may face barriers to self-care.[7,31,32] Self-efficacy is the extent or strength of one's belief in one's own ability to complete tasks and reach goals.[32] Thorough assessment and use of interventions to bridge that gap should be implemented to increase adherence to self-care. Objective data provided through telemonitoring can help patients with HF realize the cause-effect of their daily actions on their health status.[9,17]

HF education with an emphasis on self-management was the focus of multiple telemonitoring studies.[33] Although mixed outcomes were reported on the effect of HF self-care behaviors, most studies reported significant improvements including daily weighing, medication management, exercise adherence, fluid and alcohol restriction, sodium restriction, and stress reduction.[9,17]

A study comparing self-management skills using tailored telemonitoring interventions with usual care found patients in the intervention group had better knowledge of HF and increased self-care abilities and sense of self-efficacy.[17] Repetitive, tailored, disease-specific information and self-care support was individualized to the patients and addressed symptoms, knowledge, and behavior. Increased knowledge of HF and adherence to daily weight monitoring, fluid intake, activity recommendations, and importance of medication adherence was observed. Variability in initiation to sustained behavior change was noted for specific behaviors at 3, 6, and 12 months postintervention. Adherence to daily weight monitoring occurred the entire 12 months, whereas adherence to activity recommendations and medication adherence was not achieved until 3 and 6 months, respectively. Management of fluid restriction was present at 3 months and again at 12 months. No effects were found regarding appointment-keeping, diet, smoking, and use of alcohol. Researchers concluded that telemonitoring can be used to substitute some educational and self-care ability interventions performed by nurses.[17]

A highly automated and user-centered mobile phone–based telemonitoring system was used to evaluate its effect on self-care and clinical management of patients with HF.[9] The device remitted daily weight and blood pressure measurements and weekly electrocardiogram recordings. An alert message was sent to staff who monitored daily readings and the device provided patients with readings and instructions on additional interventions. Subjects had improved QOL through improved self-care and clinical management. Adherence was high and the system was feasible for all patients, including the elderly and those with no experience with mobile phones. Success was attributed to the immediate feedback patients received from clinicians familiar with their case history if potential decompensation was suspected. A subgroup analysis of study patients who received telemonitoring and were managed in the HF clinic for greater than 6 months was completed. This subgroup had significant improvements in NYHA classification, brain natriuretic peptide levels, and left ventricular function from baseline. Additional studies with larger populations are needed to assess the effects of self-care on secondary measures related to use, including emergency room visits and hospitalizations.

The importance of applying staged-based interventions to increase adherence to HF self-care has been documented in the literature.[31,32] Identifying and researching appropriate interventions specific to the management of patients with HF continues to be researched. A pilot study was conducted evaluating the preliminary effect of a motivational interviewing (MI)/transtheoretical model (TTM) intervention on HF patients' self-care behaviors.[8] The theory of heart failure self-care was used to describe the self-care process and to select the intervention.[34] The TTM of behavior change incorporates an assessment of an individual's readiness to act on a new healthier behavior, and provides strategies to guide the individual through five stages of change: (1) precontemplation, (2) contemplation, (3) preparation, (4) action, and (5) maintenance.[32] In addition to stage of change, three other major constructs are also included: (1) decisional balance (an individual's relative weighting of the pros and cons of changing),[35] (2) processes of change (how a person changes),[32] and (3) self-efficacy (confidence that a person can engage in a specific behavior).[32] The focus of MI is to assess a patient's confidence and conviction in HF self-care, which is a central factor in improving self-care and achieving behavior change.[8] The pilot results suggested that an intervention that

combines MI and TTM, as well as specifically designed intervention tools, has the potential to encourage self-care behaviors in patients with HF. Future research is needed to confirm these preliminary results. Adding technology to these concepts may enhance HF self-care management and possibly help decrease the likelihood of exacerbation.[18]

Combining telemonitoring with self-management initiatives was associated with increased HF knowledge and self-care skills that led to increased adherence to HF self-management. The effects of these interventions on hospitalization and mortality need to researched.[9]

TECHNOLOGY

Technology has evolved rapidly, and intervention designs can barely keep up. The ability to connect measurement devices to the telephone or computer using Bluetooth features is much less cumbersome than land-line telephone and hub technology currently in use at some sites, and this capability is quickly expanding.[36] Use of mobile or wearable devices to track health data is rapidly gaining momentum.[37] In one survey, US consumers reported an increased likelihood of wearing health monitoring devices (clip on pods or watches), thus it was predicted that use of wearable devices will triple in 2015.[37] Some wearable devices track activity throughout the day.[36] Trending the impact of daily activity (ie, steps taken or intensity of the activity) on heart rate or blood pressure throughout the day, versus a once-daily reading, may add valuable information on the effect of patient activity or rest and facilitate optimization of HF treatment. Many applications (apps) include trending capabilities in the form of graphs and pie charts that patients can share with the health care team during visits, or have data linked to their electronic health record.

The use of mobile phones and available apps provide a myriad of options for monitoring. Many devices/apps include tools and trackers for monitoring physical activity, diet, symptoms, and medication adherence and provide feedback of behavioral goals established by the user, social support, social comparison, prompts/cues, rewards, focus on past success, and reminders for continued use.[38] Patients with HF can be educated to use devices. Tracking and increasing activity, monitoring weight, and following dietary restrictions are all essential elements to HF care and patient education.[1,7] Validated computer algorithms are included in many mobile apps, and provide patients immediate feedback and interpretation of results.[36] Values outside of usual or preset ranges can trigger treatment recommendations.[9]

Providing purposeful and targeted intervention and feedback is important to be meaningful to patients and result in adoption of self-care practices.[18] Establishing a baseline for each patient and individualizing the alerts that reflect problem areas, along with tailored interventions, is essential to detect subtle changes in a patient's status.[18] Previous studies relied on intervention based on standardized, pre-established alerts that were monitored and responded to for additional management.[11–13] Automated detection algorithms for alerts should be available rather than relying on human judgment to account for individualization of telemonitoring use.[18]

In a review of commercially available electronic activity monitors, many included evidence-based behavior change strategies[38] that were based on patients' self-monitoring of behavior, behavioral goal setting, feedback of measured data, and discrepancy assessment between goals set and goals met.[38] Future studies should identify which behavior change strategies may be most effective. Patients may be able to become more independent and self-confident in managing their condition with technology that provides instant feedback and recommendations for immediate change through interventions and activities that are meaningful to them. Built-in behavior change strategies can make telemonitoring much more efficient and less costly, particularly if the need for clinical oversight is reduced.[17,38]

Although most mobile devices are excellent at providing direct data to individual users, the largest task for health care providers is how to effectively use patient data and the potential influx of questions requiring time and/or intervention as patients seek guidance on managing their health.[36] Identifying key data points for decision-making is essential. Telemonitoring requires new governance of responsibility, specifically related to data management, storage and archiving, accountability for the accuracy of the device, data privacy, multistate licensure, cost, and reimbursement regulations.[18] New telemedicine laws are being established by Congress and should become available in 2015.[36]

IMPLICATIONS FOR FUTURE RESEARCH

The key to the future success of telemonitoring is to identify the right HF patient population that will benefit most.[18] Studies should be designed with clear objectives that provide clinical benefit and predictive value.[18] To ascertain the potential clinical effectiveness and optimal use of telemonitoring interventions, future research should include more studies of higher methodologic quality (eg, multicenter randomized controlled trials) with a longer observation period.[11,15] New research may be challenging because of rapid development of new devices and technologies that provide immediate information to patients and their selected caregivers.

Studies that include more diverse patient populations, with HF outcomes reported for men and women and for age groups (young, middle-aged, old, and elderly) separately, should be conducted to increase the external validity of outcomes.[11,15] Selecting technology that provides multilingual capabilities may provide valuable information on the effect of technology in select ethnic groups.

Studying the effect of initiating telemonitoring earlier in the disease trajectory (NYHA class I) on health maintenance and slowing the progression of disease process may be beneficial. Identifying outcomes for subsets of patients may assist in development of a stratification model that helps identify the targeted interventions that should be applied to select groups to maximize outcomes.

Future study design should include identification of best indicators for early detection of deterioration, appropriate timing to initiate telemonitoring, how to respond to alerts, clear intent of use of the data (ie, alert management versus use of data for trending), and patient and staff barriers to using monitoring systems and data generated from them.[8] Clear definitions of broad terminology describing complimentary interventions, such as care management, DM, and videoconferencing, should be provided to ensure understanding of the full degree of scope of services provided within that delivery system to ensure outcomes can be compared.

With the influx of apps available for use with mobile phones or the Internet, selecting technology that uses fully automated systems and provides immediate feedback to patients with recommended actions to take, should increase adherence to use.[9] The assumptions that the greater the mobility of the device, the easier it is to use, should be further researched. Feedback should not only include interventions in response to alerts, such as increasing a diuretic dose or decreasing sodium intake, but also positive feedback in the form of congratulatory notes and/or additional resources to support sustained behavior change. Thus, the sustainability of use based on ease of use and positive reinforcement should be tested. Additional research is needed to assess the impact of combining select behavioral techniques, such as MI, behavior change, and self-care theory, with telemonitoring and the effect on self-care.[8,9,18,31]

The effectiveness of mobile devices with embedded evidence-based behavior change strategies should be tested.

Because lack of social support is associated with higher hospitalizations rates and mortality risk,[1] applying additional interventions to telemonitoring studies that leverage social networking concepts, such as support group sessions provided in secure chat rooms and moderated by clinical staff, should be considered. Similar strategies that were studied in cardiac rehabilitation and weight loss studies had positive outcomes.[39,40]

Studies should include a full analysis of all costs associated with telemonitoring, including costs to patients, such as additional monthly or annual subscription fees associated with accessing app use. From a health care system perspective, the cost impact on organizational and clinical routines; costs of a centralized data repository, if used; costs of data storage requirements, secure data transfer, and integration of patient information into the electronic health record; cost of staff needed to monitor and respond to alerts; and costs of informatics technology staff to troubleshoot equipment issues should be considered. In choosing electronic devices and apps for clinical research, ensure they meet coding requirements. Technology that can make staff more efficient and effective may well be cost neutral or cost-saving.[11]

SUMMARY

The use of technology to monitor patients with HF has not become part of routine care; however, telemonitoring can have a place in multidisciplinary care planning, depending on the needs, goals, and capabilities of patients. In clinical trials to date, outcomes were inconsistent in identifying the impact on hospitalization and mortality, which limit the generalizability of results. Preliminary results of studies incorporating self-care and behavior change theory with use of technology show promise, but research with large sample sizes is needed to verify results and the effects of self-care behavior change on overall hospitalization and mortality. Standard DM with telephonic coaching improved self-care results in patients with HF. Incorporating support for self-monitoring, with technology, or clinical oversight when needed, can impact self-management and QOL. Appropriately identifying patients who will most likely benefit from telemonitoring, balanced with staff effort needed to support interventions and costs of telemonitoring, are important factors that require additional research. Ultimately, it is important to learn if patients who self-monitor for

new or worsening symptoms become activated to report changes to their health care providers.

Telemonitoring should allow providers to practice at their highest skill levels, allowing multidisciplinary teams to tailor interventions and tools to meet patients' specific needs. Identifying methods to incorporate automated data into medical records benefits patient care and provides a means to study data in aggregate, to identify trends within specific populations of patients with HF that may spur development of additional HF interventions. A focus on all legal aspects of telemonitoring is essential, ensuring data are secure and patient privacy is maintained.

Additional large, randomized trials are needed before telemonitoring can be accepted as a standard of HF care. The abundance of new, portable technology that includes additional interactive features provides an opportunity to study device effectiveness in promoting monitoring and HF self-care and assess best-practice strategies. Device research should be designed to increase understanding of appropriate selection criteria matched to specific outcomes, especially reductions in hospitalizations, mortality, symptoms, and HF functional status, and improvements in self-care skill adherence, productivity, and QOL.

REFERENCES

1. Yancy C, Jessup M, Bozkurt B, et al. 2013 ACC/AHA guideline for the management of HF: a report of the American College of Cardiology Foundation/American Heart Association Task Force on Practice Guidelines. Circulation 2013;128:e240–327.
2. Weintraub A, Gregory D, Patel A, et al. A multicenter randomized controlled evaluation of automated home monitoring and telephonic disease management in patients recently hospitalized for congestive heart failure: the SPAN-CHF II trial. J Card Fail 2010; 16:285–92.
3. Dendale P, De Keulenaer G, Troisfontaines P, et al. Effect of a telemonitoring-facilitated collaboration between general practitioner and heart failure clinic on mortality and rehospilatization rates in severe heart failure: the TEMA-HF 1 (TElemonitoring in the MAnagement of Heart Failure) study. Eur J Heart Fail 2012;14:333–40.
4. Baker LC, Johnson SJ, Macaulay D, et al. Integrated telehealth and care management program for Medicare beneficiaries with chronic disease lined to savings. Health Aff 2011;30:1689–97.
5. Woodend AK, Sharrard H, Fraser M, et al. Telehome monitoring in patients with cardiac disease who are at high risk of readmission. Heart Lung 2008;37:36–45.

6. Cleland JG, Louis AA, Rigby AS, et al. Noninvasive home telemonitoring for patients with heart failure at high risk for recurrent admission and death: the Trans-European Network-Home-Care Management System (TEN-HMS) study. J Am Coll Cardiol 2005; 45:1654–64.

7. Lindenfeld J, Albert NM, Boehmer JP, et al. Executive summary: HFSA 2010 comprehensive heart failure practice guidelines. J Card Fail 2010;16: 475–539.

8. Paradis V, Cossette S, Frasure-Smith N, et al. The efficacy of a motivational nursing intervention based on the stages of change on self-care in heart failure patients. J Cardiovasc Nurs 2010;25(2):130–41.

9. Seto E, Leonard KJ, Cafazzo JA, et al. Mobile phone-based telemonitoring for heart failure management: a randomized controlled trial. J Med Internet Res 2012;14(1):e31.

10. Feltner C, Jones C, Cené C. Transitional care interventions to prevent readmissions for persons with heart failure. Ann Intern Med 2014;160:774–84.

11. Inglis SC, Clark RA, McAlister FA, et al. Structured telephone support or telemonitoring programmes for patients with chronic heart failure. The Cochrane Collaboration. Published by John Wiley & Sons, Ltd. Cochrane Database Syst Rev 2010;(8):CD007228.

12. Conway A, Inglis S, Chang A, et al. Not all systematic reviews are systematic: a meta-review of the quality of systematic reviews for non-invasive remote monitoring in heart failure. J Telemed Telecare 2013; 19(6):326–37.

13. Bashshur R, Shannon G, Smith B. The empirical foundations of telemedicine interventions for chronic disease management. Telemed J E Health 2014; 20(9):769–800.

14. Takahashi P, Pecina J, Upatising B, et al. A randomized controlled trial of telemonitoring in older adults with multiple health issues to prevent hospitalizations and emergency department visits. Arch Intern Med 2012;172:773–80.

15. Polisena J, Tran K, Cimon K. Home telemonitoring for congestive heart failure: a systematic review and meta-analysis. J Telemed Telecare 2010;16:68–76.

16. Goldberg LR, Piette JD, Walsh MN, et al. Randomized trial of a daily electronic home monitoring system in patients with advanced heart failure: the weight monitoring in heart failure (WHARF) trial. Am Heart J 2003;146:705–12.

17. Boyne JJ, Vrijhoef HJ, Spreeuwenberg M, et al. Effects of tailored telemonitoring on heart failure patients' knowledge, self-care, self-efficacy and adherence: a randomized controlled trial. Eur J Cardiovasc Nurs 2014;13(3):243–52.

18. Elwyn G, Hardisty A, Peirce S, et al. Detecting deterioration in patients with chronic disease using telemonitoring: navigating the 'trough of disillusionment'. J Eval Clin Pract 2012;18:896–903.

19. Lemay G, Azad N, Struthers C. Utilization of home telemonitoring in patients 75 years of age and over with complex heart failure. J Telemed Telecare 2013;19(1):19.

20. Fairbrother P, Ure J, Hanley J, et al. Telemonitoring for chronic HF: the views of patients and healthcare professionals – a qualitative study. J Clin Nurs 2014; 23:132–44.

21. Seto E, Leonard KJ, Cafazzo JA, et al. Perceptions and experiences of heart failure patients and clinicians on the use of mobile phone-based telemonitoring. J Med Internet Res 2012;14(1):e25.

22. Hudson L, Hamar G, Orr P, et al. Remote physiological monitoring: clinical, financial, and behavioral outcomes in a heart failure population. Dis Manag 2005;8:379–81.

23. Boyne J, Van Asselt A, Gorgels A, et al. Cost-effectiveness analysis of telemonitoring versus usual care in patients with heart failure: the TEHAF-study. J Telemed Telecare 2013;19:242–8.

24. Upatising B, Wood DL, Kremers WK, et al. Cost comparison between home telemonitoring and usual care of older adults: a randomised trial (Tele-ERA). Telemed J E Health 2014;21(1):3–8.

25. Rowan T. New grants announced to fund home telehealth systems, improve care transitions for elderly. Available at: http://www.homehealthnews.org/2010/07/new-grants-announced-to-fund-home-telehealth-systems-improve-care-transitions-for-elderly/. Accessed July 26, 2010.

26. American Telemedicine Association. Telemedicine and Telehealth Services. 2013. Available at: http://www.americantelemed.org/docs/default-source/policy/medicare-payment-of-telemedicine-and-telehealth-services.pdf. Accessed January 24, 2013.

27. Priority Health. Telemonitoring for patients with chronic conditions. 2015. Available at: http://www.priorityhealth.com/provider/manual/billing-and-payment/services/telemonitoring. Acessed November 12, 2014.

28. Priority Health. Telemonitoring services covered. 2015. Available at: http://www.priorityhealth.com/provider/manual/billing-and-payment/services/telemonitoring/services-covered. Accessed January 7, 2015.

29. Lerman A. CMS expands telehealth reimbursement in new rule. 2014. Available at: http://www.techhealthperspectives.com/telehealth-and-telemedicine/. Accessed November 5, 2014.

30. American Telemedicine Association. 2014 state telemedicine legislation tracking. Available at: http://www.americantelemed.org/docs/default-source/policy/state-telemedicine-policy-matrix.pdf?sfvrsn=70. Accessed January 31, 2014.

31. Paul S, Sneed NV. Strategies for behavior change in patients with heart failure. Am J Crit Care 2004; 13(4):305–13.

32. Prochaska JO, DiClemente CC. Stages of change in the modification of problem behaviors. Prog Behav Modif 1992;28:183–218.

33. Radhakrishnan K, Jacelon C. Impact of telehealth on patient self-management of heart failure: a review of literature. J Cardiovasc Nurs 2012;27(1):33–43.

34. Reigel B, Dickson VV. A situation-specific theory heart failure self-care. J Cardiovasc Nurs 2008;23(3):190–6.

35. Velicer WF, DiClemente CC, Prochaska JO. Decisional balance measure for assessing and predicting smoking status. J Pers Soc Psychol 1985;48(5):1279–89.

36. Topol on medicine in 2015: letting go. Medscape; 2014. Accessed December 29, 2014.

37. Auchard E. U.S. consumers warm to wearable tech, Europeans cooler-study Reuters. Available at: http://finance.yahoo.com/news/u-consumers-warm-wearable-tech-230001273.html;_ylt=A0LEVi7d.YZU8 gsAyg9jmolQ. Accessed December 8, 2014.

38. Lyons E, Lewis Z, Mayrsohn B, et al. Behavior change techniques implemented in electronic lifestyle activity monitors: a systematic content analysis. J Med Internet Res 2014;16(8):e192.

39. Forman D, LaFond K, Panch T, et al. Utility and Efficacy of smartphone application to enhance learning and behavior goals of traditional cardiac rehabilitation: a feasibility study. J Cardiopulm Rehabil Prev 2014;34:1–8.

40. Appel L, Clark J, Yeh H, et al. Comparative effectiveness of weight-loss interventions in clinical practice. N Engl J Med 2011;365(21):1959–68.

41. Chaudry S, Barton B, Curtis JP, et al. Telemonitoring in patients with heart failure. N Engl J Med 2010;363: 2301–9.

42. Koehler F, Winkler S, Shieber M, et al. Impact of remote telemedical management on mortality and hospitalizations in ambulatory patients with chronic heart failure. Circulation 2011;123:1873–80.

43. Mortara A, Pinna GD, Johnson P, et al. Home telemonitoring in heart failure patients: the HHH study (Home of Hospital in Heart Failure). European Journal of Heart Failure 2009;11:312–8.

Team-based Care for Advanced Heart Failure

Omar Wever-Pinzon, MD[a], Stavros G. Drakos, MD, PhD[b], James C. Fang, MD[b],*

KEYWORDS

- Heart failure • LVAD • Multidisciplinary team

KEY POINTS

- Advanced heart failure (AHF) is the end stage of the heart failure (HF) syndrome, with steadily increasing prevalence, significant morbidity, high mortality, and rising costs.
- Multidisciplinary team-based care of patients with AHF has been shown to reduce the risk of hospitalization, death, and health care costs in randomized controlled trials.
- Left ventricular assist devices (LVADs) have been shown to improve morbidity, mortality, quality of life, and functional capacity in patients with AHF.
- Multidisciplinary team-based care of LVAD-supported patients seems to be effective; however, supporting evidence is derived from nonrandomized studies.

INTRODUCTION

HF is an important cause of morbidity and mortality and poses a significant burden to health care systems worldwide. In the United States, over 5 million adults live with HF and 825,000 new cases are diagnosed annually.[1] HF accounts for a large proportion of medical expenditures and is now the leading cause of hospitalization in the Medicare population. Annually, more than 1 million patients are hospitalized with a primary diagnosis of HF, with half of these hospitalizations occurring in the advanced stages of the disease.[1] The prevalence of AHF has been estimated between 5% and 25% of the HF population, but data are limited.[2,3]

Advances in medical and device therapy have altered the natural history of HF by delaying the progression of the disease and improving survival, which has resulted in a growing number of patients with AHF. In general, AHF is defined as HF that is refractory to optimal medical therapy, including disease-modifying agents and cardiac resynchronization therapy.[4] Although a unified working definition for AHF is not available, diagnostic criteria and findings that can be useful in identifying patients with AHF have been described (**Box 1**).[4,5] The Interagency Registry for Mechanically Assisted Circulatory Support (INTERMACS) has developed 7 profiles that can further stratify patients with AHF, and it has been shown to correlate with outcomes after ventricular assist device implantation.[6]

The total cost for HF is estimated to be approximately 31 million per year and is projected to increase to 70 billion by 2030. Most of the expenditure is likely attributable to patients with AHF, in part due to the high rates of hospitalization, office visits, medical therapy, and indirect medical care experienced by these patients. In a recent study evaluating resource use in the last 180 days of life in Medicare beneficiaries with HF, 80% of patients were hospitalized in the last 6 months of life, with an increase in days in intensive care units and a cost increase from $28,766

The authors have no financial disclosures.

[a] Department of Medicine, Division of Cardiology, New York-Presbyterian Hospital, Columbia University Medical Center, 622 West 168th Street, New York, NY 10032, USA; [b] Department of Medicine, Division of Cardiology, University of Utah Health Sciences Center, 30 North Medical Drive, 4A100 SOM, Salt Lake City, UT 84132, USA

* Corresponding author. Division of Cardiovascular Medicine, University of Utah Health Sciences Center, 30 North Medical Drive, 4A100 SOM, Salt Lake City, UT 84132.

E-mail address: james.fang@hsc.utah.edu

Heart Failure Clin 11 (2015) 467–477
http://dx.doi.org/10.1016/j.hfc.2015.03.009
1551-7136/15/$ – see front matter © 2015 Elsevier Inc. All rights reserved.

Box 1
Diagnostic criteria and clinical events identifying patients with AHF

1. Diagnostic criteria

    a. Advanced NYHA functional class (NYHA class III-IV)

    b. Episodes of HF decompensation, characterized by either volume overload or reduced cardiac output

    c. Objective evidence of severe cardiac dysfunction shown by one of the following:

        i. LVEF less than 30%

        ii. Pseudonormal or restrictive mitral inflow pattern

        iii. PCWP greater than 16 mm Hg and/or RAP greater than 12 mm Hg

        iv. Elevated BNP or NT-proBNP plasma levels in the absence of noncardiac causes

    d. Severe impairment of functional capacity shown by one of the following:

        i. Inability to exercise

        ii. Distance walked in 6 minutes less than or equal to 300 m

        iii. Peak oxygen consumption (Vo_2) less than 12 to 14 mL/kg/min

    e. History of 1 or more HF hospitalization in the past 6 months

    f. Presence of all the previous features despite "attempts to optimize" therapy, unless these are poorly tolerated or contraindicated, and cardiac resynchronization therapy when indicated

2. Clinical events that suggest AHF

    a. Frequent (≥ 2) HF hospitalizations or ED visits in the past 12 months

    b. Progressive decline in renal function

    c. Cardiac cachexia

    d. Intolerance to ACE inhibitors because of hypotension or worsening renal function

    e. Intolerance to β-blockers because of hypotension or worsening HF

    f. Frequent systolic blood pressure less than 90 mm Hg

    g. Persistent dyspnea with dressing or bathing requiring rest

    h. Inability to walk 1 block on the level ground because of dyspnea or fatigue

    i. Escalation of diuretics to maintain euvolemia (furosemide dose >160 mg/d or use of metolazone)

    j. Progressive decline in serum sodium levels (<133 mEq/L)

    k. Frequent ICD shocks

Abbreviations: ACE, angiotensin converting enzyme; BNP, B-type natriuretic peptide; ED, emergency department; ICD, implantable cardioverter-defibrillator; LVEF, left ventricular ejection fraction; NT-proBNP, N-terminal pro-B-type natriuretic peptide; NYHA, New York Heart Association; PWCP, pulmonary capillary wedge pressure; RAP, right atrial pressure; Vo_2, oxygen consumption.

Adapted from Yancy CW, Jessup M, Bozkurt B, et al. 2013 ACCF/AHA guideline for the management of heart failure: a report of the American College of Cardiology Foundation/American Heart Association Task Force on practice guidelines. Circulation 2013;128(16):e240–327; and Metra M, Ponikowski P, Dickstein K, et al. Advanced chronic heart failure: a position statement from the Study Group on Advanced Heart Failure of the Heart Failure Association of the European Society of Cardiology. Eur J Heart Fail 2007;9(6–7):684–94, with permission.

to $36,216 per patient.[7] Recent data on the comparative cost-effectiveness of advanced therapies for this group of patients suggest that although heart transplant is a life-prolonging and cost-effective therapy, the use of long-term mechanical circulatory support requires additional improvement in its adverse event profile and quality of life to reach an acceptable cost-effectiveness threshold.[8]

Thus, the growing number of patients with AHF in conjunction with the high complexity of their management and rising health care costs requires the development and implementation of health care models that allow for optimal and comprehensive management of these patients, while taking into consideration the limitations imposed by the health care system. A multidisciplinary team-based approach has been proposed to improve staff communication, patient outcomes, and satisfaction as well as reduce length of hospital stay and hospitalization rates.[9]

IMPACT OF TEAM-BASED CARE IN ADVANCED HEART FAILURE

The primary goal of multidisciplinary HF management programs is to improve patient survival and quality of life (**Box 2**). Multiple randomized controlled trials have been conducted in recent years comparing a multidisciplinary team-based approach with usual care of patients with HF and show consistent results. Multidisciplinary

---

Box 2
Impact of team-based care in AHF

1. Goals

   a. Reduce morbidity

      i. Symptom control

      ii. Improve quality of life

      iii. Improve exercise capacity

      iv. Reduce readmissions

      v. Establish patient's end-of-life goals

   b. Reduce mortality

2. Strategies

   a. Early recognition of signs and symptoms of HF decompensation

   b. Improve adherence to guideline-directed medical and device-based therapy

   c. Achievement of effective doses of disease-modifying pharmacologic agents

   d. Exercise training

   e. Advanced interventions

      i. Heart transplant

      ii. Temporary or long-term mechanical circulatory support

      iii. Investigational surgical and pharmacologic options

      iv. Palliative care and hospice

         1. Long-term inotropic support

         2. ICD deactivation

Abbreviation: ICD, implantable cardioverter-defibrillator.

---

strategies reduce mortality by 25% to 46%, HF hospitalizations by 25%, and all-cause hospitalizations by 20% to 30%.[9,10] Furthermore, multidisciplinary HF management programs have demonstrated to reduce length of stay and improve quality of life scores compared with usual care.[11,12] The observed improvement in outcomes can be attributed to greater adherence to guideline-directed medical therapies, higher proportion of patients achieving effective doses of disease-modifying pharmacologic agents, and early recognition of signs and symptoms of HF decompensation.[13,14] As a result of the clear benefits of multidisciplinary team-based HF management programs, the development and enrollment of patients with AHF in such programs is given the highest level of recommendation by current clinical practice guidelines.[4] However, most trials have included a variable degree of HF severity, and trials that specifically address the AHF population are limited.

STRUCTURE OF THE MULTIDISCIPLINARY TEAM-BASED HEART FAILURE MANAGEMENT PROGRAM

A multidisciplinary HF team is formed by a group of medical and nonmedical personnel who participate in the care of patients with HF and communicate regularly and effectively with each other with the primary goal of improving patient outcomes and satisfaction, while reducing health care costs. The team-based care of patients with AHF is typically led by HF cardiologists, in conjunction with dedicated nursing staff, pharmacists, nutritionists, physical therapists, social workers, and case managers (**Fig. 1**). The complementary role of the additional team members allows patients with AHF to receive a higher number and quality of services, such as counseling on behavioral change or self-management support, which are often outside the expertise of the HF cardiologist (**Table 1**).

Patient Referral and Initial Evaluation

Patients with HF who may benefit from being managed by a multidisciplinary team are often referred at the time of HF hospitalization discharge or by a care provider who identifies a patient at increased risk for negative outcomes (see **Fig. 1**). The first step in the evaluation of these patients is to determine whether or not they have AHF. This task can be accomplished by excluding alternative causes of advanced symptoms and by means of the diagnostic criteria and high-risk features previously described. The multidisciplinary team should perform a comprehensive evaluation

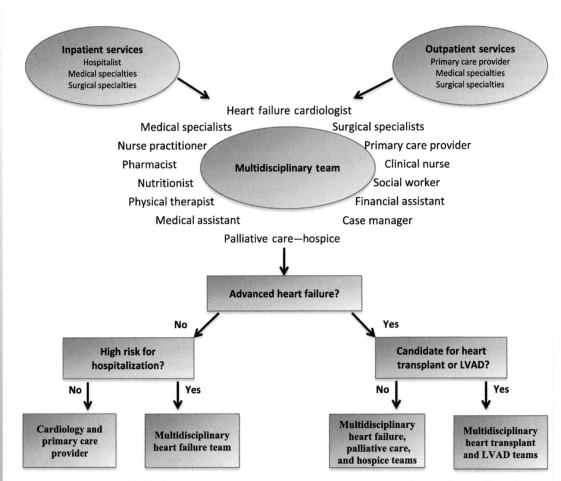

Fig. 1. Structure of multidisciplinary team and goal-based algorithm management of patients with AHF.

for the adequacy and maximization of pharmacologic therapy, cardiac resynchronization therapy, and treatment of reversible causes of myocardial dysfunction (eg, hemodynamically significant coronary artery disease) as indicated. Other considerations include hemodynamic assessment if appropriate, role of cardiotoxic agents for other conditions (eg, chemotherapy), treatment of comorbid conditions, as well as review of end-organ function, pulmonary hypertension, and other conditions that would preclude the use of AHF therapies, that is, heart transplant and mechanical circulatory support.

Comprehensive Evaluation

An important aspect of the comprehensive assessment of these patients is psychosocial evaluation, because psychosocial issues such as depression and lack of social support are linked to reduced compliance with medical therapy and poor clinical outcomes including fatal and nonfatal cardiovascular events.[15,16] Furthermore, there is inadequate health literacy in 27% to 44% of adults older than 65 years. Thus, it is important to identify patients' psychosocial issues, evaluate their living environment, and identify a reliable primary caregiver. Another component of the evaluation involves the assessment of quality of life through validated measures and questionnaires that will set a baseline status for each patient and will be used as an outcome measure of the therapeutic interventions implemented by the team. Patients with AHF have multiple comorbidities, such as malnutrition, anemia, depression, renal insufficiency, and chronic pulmonary disease that often require evaluation by different specialists (nutritionists, psychiatrists, pulmonologists, and nephrologists). The participation of other specialists in the multidisciplinary team, in consultative and educational roles, allows for early recognition, management, and close follow-up, which contribute to better outcomes.

Goal-Oriented Team-based Care

Based on the initial comprehensive assessment and patient preferences, a treatment plan should

Table 1
Role of team members caring for patients with AHF

Providers	Responsible for clinical aspects of care
HF cardiologist	• Team leader and clinical decision maker • Patient and family educator • Identifies reversible causes of myocardial dysfunction • Maximizes pharmacotherapy and CRT±D • Timely involvement of appropriate consultants • Candidate selection for advanced therapies

Medical specialists	• Advice in specialized aspects of care, including the evaluation and treatment of comorbidities such as:
	  ◦ Psychiatric disorders
	  ◦ Renal insufficiency
	  ◦ Pulmonary disease
	  ◦ Malignancy
	  ◦ Neurologic disorders and anoxic brain injury in patients with cardiac arrest
	  ◦ Device (defibrillator or CRT) infections

Surgical specialists	• Provide specialized care including:
	  ◦ High-risk valvular and CABG surgery
	  ◦ Myectomy
	  ◦ Ablation procedures for atrial and ventricular arrhythmias
	  ◦ Epicardial lead placement for CRT±D
	  ◦ Mechanical circulatory support
	  ◦ Noncardiac surgical procedures

Palliative care—hospice	• Establish an end-of-life plan of care • Support individual and family needs • ICD deactivation • Prevent and treat discomfort or pain
Primary care provider	• Point of first contact, responsible for early referral • Continuous care of cardiac and noncardiac conditions in close collaboration with team
Nurse practitioner	• Provide direct clinical care • Patient and family educator • Maximization of pharmacologic and device therapy
Allied health professionals	**Enhance, support, and expand providers' services**
Pharmacist	• Monitor for appropriateness of medical regimen and possible drug-drug interaction • Suggest approaches to continue effective medical therapy while minimizing side effects
Nutritionist	• Expert advice on nutritional support and supplementation
Physical therapist	• Evaluates patient's physical limitations and disabilities • Promotes mobility and improvement in functional capacity by different physical interventions
Medical assistant	• Perform a wide array of administrative and clinical duties that support provider services
Case manager	• Coordination of the efforts of individual team members. Advocate for patients and their families by coordinating care and linking the patient with the team, resources, and payers • Coordination of medical and nonmedical services
Financial assistant/coordinator	• Deals with the economic aspects of health care and facilitates patient's access to care (particularly important for advanced therapies) and provider's reimbursement
Social worker	• Aid patients and family to address social problems (eg, help in dealing with prolonged absence from work and possible job loss) • Counseling and psychotherapy
Clinical nurse	• Delivers specific services and support • Provides the substance and structure of the entire caring process itself

Abbreviations: CABG, coronary artery bypass graft; CRT, cardiac resynchronization therapy; CRT±D, cardiac resynchronization therapy +/− defibrillator; ICD, implantable cardioverter-defibrillator.

be formulated. If patients are deemed to be adequate candidates for heart transplant or long-term mechanical circulatory support, they are evaluated by the multidisciplinary heart transplant and/or LVAD teams. In patients with AHF who do not require immediate referral for heart transplant or LVAD implantation, or in patients who are ineligible for these advanced therapies, a treatment plan that involves close monitoring and early involvement of palliative care services for the latter should be formulated. It is important to keep in mind that independent of the treatment plan, the team should continue to work in close liaison with the referring primary care provider and/or referring cardiologist. The use of the shared care model by the multidisciplinary team allows providing advanced care to patients living in remote areas, while maintaining the patients in their own community, which translates to improved quality of life and outcomes. A successful model should constantly communicate and collaborate with the referring provider by offering education and expert clinical support, sharing educational material and disease management protocols, and designing expedited venues to address adverse events that require prompt evaluation and management by the advanced multidisciplinary team.

MONITORING OF PATIENTS WITH ADVANCED HEART FAILURE

Monitoring of patients with AHF depends on the clinical condition of the patient and the treatment plan established by the multidisciplinary team. The immediate priority is to maintain physiologic stability and to reestablish euvolemia and adequate perfusion in patients evaluated during an acute decompensation. In patients with AHF, similar to patients with less-advanced stages of the disease, education to facilitate HF self-care and self-management, sodium restriction, and exercise training is recommended.[4] Furthermore, optimization of pharmacologic therapy should be attempted whenever possible, as tolerated based on symptoms, end-organ perfusion, and electrolyte levels. The addition of B-type natriuretic peptide (BNP) or N-terminal pro-BNP (NT-proBNP) to multidisciplinary care to guide medical therapy has yielded conflicting results. BNP or NT-proBNP is recommended as a prognostic marker for risk stratification purposes, and their trajectory may be useful to follow-up patients who are challenging historians.

Close monitoring of patients with AHF allows the multidisciplinary team to identify early signs and symptoms of volume overload and/or clinical deterioration and end-organ dysfunction. In patients with evidence of volume overload, diuretics and sodium restriction are indicated to relieve congestive symptoms. If diuretic resistance develops, a combination of diuretics with different mechanisms of action (eg, loop and thiazide diuretics) can be used, while frequently monitoring levels of serum electrolytes and renal function. In case of volume overload refractory to a combination of diuretics or in the presence of worsening renal function, consultation with a nephrologist may be appropriate to evaluate renal replacement therapies.

In patients presenting with cardiogenic shock or signs of hypoperfusion with end-organ dysfunction, the use of positive inotropic agents is recommended as a temporizing measure until myocardial function recovers or a heart transplant or LVAD implantation occurs. Inotrope-dependent patients (INTERMACS 1–3) require prompt evaluation by the multidisciplinary team for heart transplant and LVAD therapy. Patients ineligible for LVAD therapy or heart transplant should be referred to the palliative care arm of the multidisciplinary team. Avoiding late referral for advanced therapies is a critical aspect of a multidisciplinary team, because outcomes of advanced therapies will be optimal if the patient has not deteriorated to the point where surgical morbidity and mortality are prohibitive.

PALLIATIVE CARE OF PATIENTS WITH ADVANCED HEART FAILURE

An important and challenging aspect of the team-based care of patients with AHF is the early recognition of the terminal stages of the disease and timely involvement of palliative care services. The multidisciplinary team should discuss with the patient and caregivers the patient's prognosis and treatment options. The team should establish an end-of-life plan of care with the primary objective of preventing and treating discomfort or pain, support patient's needs, and prioritize patient's quality of life. In order to accomplish this task, an adequate communication with the palliative care and hospice teams that involves feedback on patient's condition is essential.[17] Arrhythmias are common at the end of life and a particularly vexing issue to reconcile. Patients who have an implantable cardioverter defibrillator, however, may be denied the opportunity of a sudden cardiac death, and instead are committed to a slow terminal decline, with frequent and painful device shocks that can decrease their quality of life, greatly contributing to their distress and that of their families during this period. Therefore, deactivation of the implantable cardioverter-defibrillator should be addressed, as supported by current guidelines.

TEAM-BASED CARE OF LEFT VENTRICULAR ASSIST DEVICE SUPPORTED PATIENTS
Team-based Care at the Time of Left Ventricular Assist Device Implantation

The observed improvement in survival in the Randomized Evaluation of Mechanical Assistance for the Treatment of Congestive Heart Failure (REMATCH) trial over time has been attributed to infection prevention and nutritional protocols derived using a multidisciplinary approach and this ultimately led to a reduction in sepsis, device-related infections, renal failure, and a trend toward fewer bleeding complications in patients enrolled in the second half of the trial.[18] The Utah Artificial Heart Program/Utah Transplant Affiliated Hospitals (UTAH) Cardiac Transplant Program, the highest enrolling center for the REMATCH trial, used a multidisciplinary approach throughout their involvement in the trial; this program experienced a 38% lower rate of adverse events and higher 1-year survival in the Utah cohort (77%) compared with the rest of the REMATCH trial (52%).[19]

Team-based care (**Fig. 2**) of LVAD recipients should begin during the preimplantation phase. This approach improves the evaluation of LVAD candidates and especially helps to identify psychosocial factors that might jeopardize outcomes. In addition, nutritional assessment by a registered dietician, pharmacist, and a physician (with specialized nutrition support training) is critical to assessing the candidate's ability to undergo the rigors of major cardiac surgery. Different nutritional assessment tools, macronutrient requirement estimation, and replenishment protocols based on nutritional risk have been previously described in LVAD-supported patients.[20] Coordinators and other team members provide patient and caregiver education, which improves the informed consent process and patient satisfaction.

After LVAD placement, these patients are taken care of in the intensive care unit by nursing staff, intensivists, cardiothoracic surgeons, HF cardiologists, respiratory therapists, pharmacists, nutritionists, as well as speech pathology and physical therapists. The early postoperative period focuses on maintaining hemodynamic (from bleeding or vasoplegia) and respiratory compensation, while monitoring closely for signs of right ventricular failure. Once hemodynamically stable and without significant metabolic disturbance, the patients are weaned from mechanical ventilation and vasoactive support and LVAD function is further optimized. Over the following days, the patients continue to work with the nutritionists, physical therapists, pharmacists, LVAD coordinators, and social work teams to meet the nutritional requirements; transition to a more independent functional status; become proficient in the management of LVAD, driveline care, and medical regimen; and reintegrate to the community.

Half of the patients are discharged to acute inpatient rehabilitation after LVAD implantation.[21] After 7 to 12 days in the inpatient rehabilitation unit, most patients experience a positive change in their functional status, with an increment in their mean total Functional Independence Measure scale score of 18 to 22 points.[21,22]

Team-based Care of Long-term Left Ventricular Assist Device Support

Implications of team-based care on long-term left ventricular assist device support
The accelerated increase in the number of implanting centers and patients receiving an LVAD,[6] along with mounting efforts to maximize efficiency and limit unnecessary consumption of health care resources, has brought into question the cost-effectiveness of this therapy.[23] The costs associated with LVAD therapy include those related to LVAD implant hospitalization, costs related to complications after LVAD implantation, and costs related to heart transplant in eligible patients. Readmissions are common in LVAD-supported patients and negatively impact survival, as it has been recently shown.[24] Furthermore, avoidance of complications after LVAD implantation could improve their cost-effectiveness by 40% to 50%, that is, a bridge to transplant (BTT)-LVAD would cost $128,000 versus $226,000 per quality-adjusted life-year (QALY) gained and a destination therapy (DT)-LVAD would cost $100,000 versus $202,000 per QALY gained if medical complications occurred.[8] A team-based approach has the potential to decrease costs associated with the index hospitalization as well as costs after LVAD implantation. Institution of a multidisciplinary team resulted in reduced length of stay, 30-day readmission rate, and post-LVAD cost, compared with a system based on a single discipline (cardiac surgery).[25] The focus of the care by the multidisciplinary team in the chronic phase of LVAD support (see **Fig. 2**) is to provide continuous education and support to patients and caregivers, with emphasis on driveline care and compliance with complex medical regimens. Furthermore, LVAD recipients often face complex psychological and emotional problems and, although the quality of life improves after LVAD implantation, significant depression and anxiety remain a problem in up to 36% of

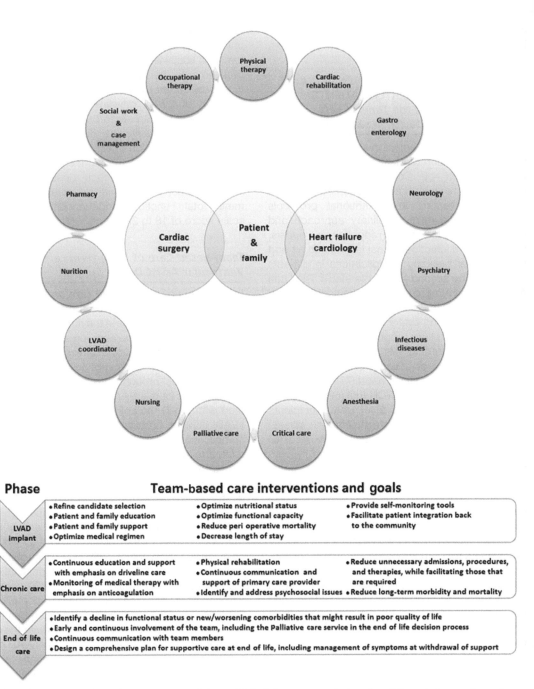

Fig. 2. Structure, goals, and interventions of the multidisciplinary team during the different phases of care in patients with ventricular assist devices.

patients.[26] Taking this fact into consideration, the members of the team should promptly identify psychological problems that may ensue in LVAD recipients and refer the patient for psychiatric evaluation. Enrollment in a cardiac rehabilitation program is of utmost importance because it can potentially improve functional capacity, quality of life, and depression among LVAD recipients.[27]

Some patients may live far away from the implant center, therefore most of the direct patient care and LVAD support is provided by the local primary care provider. It is then of paramount importance that the implanting team remains in regular contact with the patient and assumes the following responsibilities: provide continuous LVAD education and support to the primary care provider and local services, monitor the device function periodically, and provide supplies required for the appropriate functioning and monitoring of the pump.

Team-based care of left ventricular assist device-related adverse events

Bleeding is the most frequent adverse event associated with continuous-flow LVAD support, with rates of 1.4 events per patient-year in the BTT population and 0.9 events per patient-year in patients undergoing destination therapy.[28,29] The bleeding diathesis observed in LVAD recipients is multifactorial and has been attributed to factors such as anticoagulation, acquired von Willebrand syndrome, and reduced pulsatility.[30,31] Gastrointestinal bleeding is the most common cause of nonsurgical bleeding in patients supported by continuous-flow LVADs.[31,32] A team-based approach, with team members familiarized with the mechanisms of bleeding in this population, is essential to manage bleeding complications. Gastroenterologists familiar with this patient population are more likely to elect testing and therapeutic options that would result in bleeding resolution successfully.

A complication that has recently gained public attention is the occurrence of LVAD thrombosis because reports indicate an increase in its incidence 3 months postimplant, from 2.2% to 8.4% after March 2011.[33] This increase in incidence has been attributed to changes in anticoagulation strategies over time in an attempt to diminish bleeding complications. In this regard, a multidisciplinary approach that involves a pharmacist-managed international normalized ratio with patient self-testing resulted in a greater percentage time in therapeutic range of the international normalized ratio compared with usual care (44% vs 31%, $P = .03$), which might translate into decreased rates of pump thrombosis in large cohorts of patients. Furthermore, patients with prior hematologic conditions are at high risk for bleeding, thrombotic and neurologic complications, and increased mortality after LVAD implantation.[34] Thus, consultation with a hematologist familiar with LVADs is reasonable and may potentially translate into better outcomes. Neurologic complications, including intracranial hemorrhage (0.01–0.05 events per patient-years)[28,29] and ischemic cerebrovascular accident (0.03–0.06 events per patient-years)[28,29] are dreaded complications of LVAD therapy. A multidisciplinary approach to these complications with a dedicated neurology team familiar with the management of LVAD-supported patients has been recently described,[35] although whether this approach improves outcomes is unknown.

LVAD-related infections represent a significant cause of morbidity and mortality in patients supported with LVADs. Multidisciplinary approaches directed at preventing and treating infectious complications during LVAD support have been previously described,[36] which in the authors' experience has resulted in improved outcomes.

As the number of patients on LVAD support continues to grow, multidisciplinary teams are now facing an increasing number of non-LVAD-related adverse events. These noncardiac complications often require interventions that range from dental extraction to hip replacement and abdominal surgery.[37,38] Inclusion of surgical specialists experienced in the management of LVAD-supported patients would result in unnecessary delays and unnecessary procedures and may result in reduced perioperative bleeding.

TEAM-BASED CARE AND END OF LIFE IN LEFT VENTRICULAR ASSIST DEVICE SUPPORTED PATIENTS

Patients supported with LVADs, particularly those implanted as a destination therapy, eventually face the end of life with their device in place. The presence of an implanted device that must be turned off can bring major ethical concerns, distress, and confusion for the unprepared health care provider, patient, and caregiver. In response to these concerns, a multidisciplinary team-based approach with palliative medicine consultation has shown to improve end-of-life care by focusing on improved communication, patient and caregiver support, quality of life, and symptom management. Brush and colleagues[39] reported the experience of the multidisciplinary team at the Utah Artificial Heart Program/UTAH Cardiac Transplant Program in dealing with the end of life in patients receiving an LVAD as a destination therapy. This experience revealed that LVAD deactivation and end-of-life discussions were typically brought up when quality of life for the LVAD-supported patient was no longer acceptable, either because of progressive decline in functional capacity and cognition or worsening comorbidities. Tasks of the multidisciplinary team that were key elements in improving patient and family satisfaction included acknowledgment and support of the patient's decision to terminate LVAD support, design of a detailed plan and active participation during the pump deactivation process, as well as early palliative care involvement for supportive care and symptom relief. Although different algorithms to facilitate preparation of the multidisciplinary team for LVAD deactivation have been proposed,[40,41] the fundamental elements of a team-based care of LVAD-supported patients at the end of life include an effective communication with the patient, family, and among teams; palliative care consultation; and coordination of multidisciplinary care at the bedside.

SUMMARY

A multidisciplinary team-based approach to the care of patients with HF has shown in multiple randomized controlled trials to improve patient outcomes and is therefore recommended by current guidelines as a management strategy across the wide spectrum of stages in the HF syndrome. A team-based care of patients with AHF is more likely to be successful in establishing a plan of care to maintain stability and also to promptly identify clinical deterioration that will require a change in the plan of care, incorporating heart transplant, mechanical support, and/or palliative care services to the treatment plan. The team-based care of LVAD-supported patients seems to derive similar benefits to the ones observed in the management of HF; however, randomized studies are required to evaluate the effectiveness of this intervention in this particular population.

Successful multidisciplinary teams have typically included HF cardiologists, cardiothoracic surgeons, nursing staff, social workers, case managers, pharmacists, nutritionists, and physical therapists, and this allows for a comprehensive coordination of care across the variety of health and social needs of the patients. Incorporation of other specialties to the multidisciplinary team is appropriate because these patients typically have several comorbidities such as cognitive impairment, depression, renal insufficiency, respiratory disorders, and anemia that may benefit from specialized evaluation as considered appropriate. Participation of specialists in palliative care in the multidisciplinary team is a fundamental component of effective end-of-life care, and their input will unquestionably enhance patient comfort, facilitate better access to hospice care, and promote advance care planning.

REFERENCES

1. Go AS, Mozaffarian D, Roger VL, et al. Heart disease and stroke statistics–2014 update: a report from the American Heart Association. Circulation 2014;129(3):e28–292.
2. Nohria A, Lewis E, Stevenson LW. Medical management of advanced heart failure. JAMA 2002;287(5): 628–40.
3. Adams KF Jr, Zannad F. Clinical definition and epidemiology of advanced heart failure. Am Heart J 1998;135(6 Pt 2 Su):S204–15.
4. Yancy CW, Jessup M, Bozkurt B, et al. 2013 ACCF/AHA guideline for the management of heart failure: a report of the American College of Cardiology Foundation/American Heart Association Task Force on practice guidelines. Circulation 2013;128(16): e240–327.
5. Metra M, Ponikowski P, Dickstein K, et al. Advanced chronic heart failure: a position statement from the Study Group on Advanced Heart Failure of the Heart Failure Association of the European Society of Cardiology. Eur J Heart Fail 2007;9(6–7):684–94.
6. Kirklin JK, Naftel DC, Pagani FD, et al. Sixth INTERMACS annual report: a 10,000-patient database. J Heart Lung Transpl 2014;33(6):555–64.
7. Unroe KT, Greiner MA, Hernandez AF, et al. Resource use in the last 6 months of life among Medicare beneficiaries with heart failure, 2000–2007. Arch Intern Med 2011;171(3):196–203.
8. Long EF, Swain GW, Mangi AA. Comparative survival and cost-effectiveness of advanced therapies for end-stage heart failure. Circ Heart Fail 2014; 7(3):470–8.
9. McAlister FA, Stewart S, Ferrua S, et al. Multidisciplinary strategies for the management of heart failure patients at high risk for admission: a systematic review of randomized trials. J Am Coll Cardiol 2004;44(4):810–9.
10. Feltner C, Jones CD, Cene CW, et al. Transitional care interventions to prevent readmissions for persons with heart failure: a systematic review and meta-analysis. Ann Intern Med 2014;160(11): 774–84.
11. White SM, Hill A. A heart failure initiative to reduce the length of stay and readmission rates. Prof Case Manag 2014;19(6):276–84.
12. Kasper EK, Gerstenblith G, Hefter G, et al. A randomized trial of the efficacy of multidisciplinary care in heart failure outpatients at high risk of hospital readmission. J Am Coll Cardiol 2002;39(3):471–80.
13. Rich MW, Gray DB, Beckham V, et al. Effect of a multidisciplinary intervention on medication compliance in elderly patients with congestive heart failure. Am J Med 1996;101(3):270–6.
14. McDonald K, Ledwidge M, Cahill J, et al. Elimination of early rehospitalization in a randomized, controlled trial of multidisciplinary care in a high-risk, elderly heart failure population: the potential contributions of specialist care, clinical stability and optimal angiotensin-converting enzyme inhibitor dose at discharge. Eur J Heart Fail 2001;3(2):209–15.
15. Richardson LG. Psychosocial issues in patients with congestive heart failure. Prog Cardiovasc Nurs 2003;18(1):19–27.

16. Krumholz HM, Butler J, Miller J, et al. Prognostic importance of emotional support for elderly patients hospitalized with heart failure. Circulation 1998; 97(10):958–64.

17. Jaarsma T, Beattie JM, Ryder M, et al. Palliative care in heart failure: a position statement from the palliative care workshop of the Heart Failure Association of the European Society of Cardiology. Eur J Heart Fail 2009;11(5):433–43.

18. Park SJ, Tector A, Piccioni W, et al. Left ventricular assist devices as destination therapy: a new look at survival. J Thorac Cardiovasc Surg 2005;129(1):9–17.

19. Long JW, Healy AH, Rasmusson BY, et al. Improving outcomes with long-term "destination" therapy using left ventricular assist devices. J Thorac Cardiovasc Surg 2008;135(6):1353–60 [discussion: 1360–1].

20. Holdy K, Dembitsky W, Eaton LL, et al. Nutrition assessment and management of left ventricular assist device patients. J Heart Lung Transpl 2005; 24(10):1690–6.

21. Alsara O, Reeves RK, Pyfferoen MD, et al. Inpatient rehabilitation outcomes for patients receiving left ventricular assist device. Am J Phys Med Rehabil 2014;93(10):860–8.

22. English ML, Speed J. Effectiveness of acute inpatient rehabilitation after left ventricular assist device placement. Am J Phys Med Rehabil 2013;92(7): 621–6.

23. Moreno SG, Novielli N, Cooper NJ. Cost-effectiveness of the implantable HeartMate II left ventricular assist device for patients awaiting heart transplantation. J Heart Lung Transplant 2012;31(5):450–8.

24. Smedira NG, Hoercher KJ, Lima B, et al. Unplanned hospital readmissions after HeartMate II implantation: frequency, risk factors, and impact on resource use and survival. JACC Heart Fail 2013;1(1):31–9.

25. Murray MA, Osaki S, Edwards NM, et al. Multidisciplinary approach decreases length of stay and reduces cost for ventricular assist device therapy. Interact Cardiovasc Thorac Surg 2009;8(1):84–8.

26. Modica M, Ferratini M, Torri A, et al. Quality of life and emotional distress early after left ventricular assist device implant: a mixed-method study. Artif Organs 2015;39(3):220–7.

27. Karapolat H, Engin C, Eroglu M, et al. Efficacy of the cardiac rehabilitation program in patients with end-stage heart failure, heart transplant patients, and left ventricular assist device recipients. Transplant Proc 2013;45(9):3381–5.

28. Starling RC, Naka Y, Boyle AJ, et al. Results of the post-U.S. Food and Drug Administration-approval study with a continuous flow left ventricular assist device as a bridge to heart transplantation: a prospective study using the INTERMACS (Interagency

29. Jorde UP, Kushwaha SS, Tatooles AJ, et al. Results of the destination therapy post-food and drug administration approval study with a continuous flow left ventricular assist device: a prospective study using the INTERMACS registry (Interagency Registry for Mechanically Assisted Circulatory Support). J Am Coll Cardiol 2014;63(17):1751–7.

30. Crow S, Chen D, Milano C, et al. Acquired von Willebrand syndrome in continuous-flow ventricular assist device recipients. Ann Thorac Surg 2010; 90(4):1263–9 [discussion: 1269].

31. Wever-Pinzon O, Selzman CH, Drakos SG, et al. Pulsatility and the risk of nonsurgical bleeding in patients supported with the continuous-flow left ventricular assist device HeartMate II. Circ Heart Fail 2013;6(3):517–26.

32. Kushnir VM, Sharma S, Ewald GA, et al. Evaluation of GI bleeding after implantation of left ventricular assist device. Gastrointest Endosc 2012;75(5):973–9.

33. Starling RC, Moazami N, Silvestry SC, et al. Unexpected abrupt increase in left ventricular assist device thrombosis. N Engl J Med 2014;370(1):33–40.

34. Fried J, Levin AP, Mody KM, et al. Prior hematologic conditions carry a high morbidity and mortality in patients supported with continuous-flow left ventricular assist devices. J Heart Lung Transplant 2014; 33(11):1119–25.

35. Willey JZ, Demmer RT, Takayama H, et al. Cerebrovascular disease in the era of left ventricular assist devices with continuous flow: risk factors, diagnosis, and treatment. J Heart Lung Transplant 2014;33(9): 878–87.

36. Wever-Pinzon O, Stehlik J, Kfoury AG, et al. Ventricular assist devices: pharmacological aspects of a mechanical therapy. Pharmacol Ther 2012;134(2):189–99.

37. Taghavi S, Beyer C, Vora H, et al. Non-cardiac Surgery in patients on mechanical circulatory support. ASAIO J 2014;60(6):670–4.

38. Gogas BD, Parissis JT, Filippatos GS, et al. Severe anaemia and subcapital femur fracture in a patient with Left Ventricular Assist Device Heart Mate II: the cardiologist's management of this rare patient. Eur J Heart Fail 2009;11(8):806–8.

39. Brush S, Budge D, Alharethi R, et al. End-of-life decision making and implementation in recipients of a destination left ventricular assist device. J Heart Lung Transplant 2010;29(12):1337–41.

40. Schaefer KG, Griffin L, Smith C, et al. An interdisciplinary checklist for left ventricular assist device deactivation. J Palliat Med 2014;17(1):4–5.

41. Gafford EF, Luckhardt AJ, Swetz KM. Deactivation of a left ventricular assist device at the end of life #269. J Palliat Med 2013;16(8):980–2.

Team-based Palliative and End-of-life Care for Heart Failure

Timothy J. Fendler, MD, MS[a],*, Keith M. Swetz, MD, MA[b],
Larry A. Allen, MD, MHS[c]

KEYWORDS

- Palliative care • Hospice care • Heart failure • Interdisciplinary communication • Patient care team
- Comprehensive health care

KEY POINTS

- Palliative care is one component of holistic, supportive care of patients throughout the course of disease, intensified at end of life and extending into the bereavement phase for their caregivers.
- Team-based palliative care for heart failure implies a multidisciplinary approach, including primary care, cardiology, and palliative care, each represented by various providers (eg, physicians, advanced practitioners, nurses, case managers, and pharmacists).
- Patients require a heart failure medical home, where various specialties may take a more central role in coordination of patient care at different times in the disease span, sometimes with consultation by palliative care and sometimes transitioning focus to palliative care at the end of life.

INTRODUCTION

Among an estimated 5.1 million Americans with heart failure, the prevalence of advanced disease is 5% to 10%.[1] As such, nearly half a million Americans struggle with significant symptom burden, psychosocial stressors, and difficult decisions imposed by their end-stage heart failure. Disease prevalence is expected to grow 25% by 2030, primarily because of improved survival, whereas costs are projected to increase from $32 billion in 2013 to $70 billion in 2030.[1] With increased emphasis on patient-centered care,[2,3] and in response to unsustainable health care expenditures, there has been increasing attention placed on palliative and end-of-life care for patients with advanced heart failure.[4]

The 2013 American College of Cardiology Foundation (ACCF)/American Heart Association (AHA) guidelines support the use of palliative care in patients with end-stage heart failure as level 1B.[4] Medicare's 2014 update to National Coverage Determination for mechanical circulatory support (MCS) even mandates a multidisciplinary team that includes a palliative care specialist.[5] However, there is limited evidence to guide the content, implementation of, and integration of palliative care interventions into existing heart failure disease management. Therefore, this article explores evidence supporting a team-based approach to palliative and end-of-life care for patients with heart failure, comments on the current state of multidisciplinary care for such patients, identifies

Disclosures: Dr T.J. Fendler is supported by a T32 grant from the NHLBI (T32HL110837); the other coauthors have no relevant disclosures or potential conflicts of interest.
[a] Division of Cardiovascular Outcomes Research, Saint Luke's Mid America Heart Institute, University of Missouri-Kansas City School of Medicine, 4401 Wornall Road, SLNI, CV Research, Suite 5603, Kansas City, MO 64111, USA; [b] Section of Palliative Medicine, Division of General Internal Medicine, Department of Medicine, Mayo Clinic, 200 1st St SW, Rochester, MN 55905, USA; [c] Division of Cardiology, Department of Medicine, University of Colorado School of Medicine, 12605 East 16th Avenue, 3rd Floor, Aurora, CO 80045, USA
* Corresponding author.
E-mail address: fendlert@umkc.edu

Heart Failure Clin 11 (2015) 479–498
http://dx.doi.org/10.1016/j.hfc.2015.03.010

heartfailure.theclinics.com

knowledge gaps, and discusses opportunities for future study.

Team-based Care Implies a Multidisciplinary Approach

Ample evidence shows that team-based care for patients with heart failure decreases rehospitalizations and improves survival through education, structured follow-up, patient self-care, and care-plan adherence.[6,7] However, few pilot studies have assessed the efficacy of multidisciplinary palliative care in improving outcomes germane to end-stage heart failure (ie, quality of life, symptom control, decreased health care use, lower financial and caregiver burdens), in part because of heterogeneity in defining what palliative care is and how it should be delivered. **Table 1** details selected clinical trials and intervention studies that support a multidisciplinary palliative approach by incorporating specialties tailored to patient needs to facilitate the inevitable transitions in chronic heart failure care.

What's in a Name? Palliative Care is Supportive Care

Historically, the term palliative care was conflated with hospice care: a focused approach to dying patients for whom disease-targeted treatment or cure is no longer viable. However, this narrow restriction has given way to a more holistic view of disease management in which supportive care is afforded to all patients with chronic or life-threatening illness (**Fig. 1**). Optimal palliative care ideally begins early in the course of the disease and continues in parallel with heart failure–targeted therapy in an integrative, multidisciplinary manner.[20–22] All health care providers should strive to treat the whole patient collaboratively with a team of colleagues. Likewise, heart failure clinicians should maintain concurrent foci on treating disease, extending survival, and optimizing quality of life for patients with chronic heart failure at all disease stages.

Building on Experience or Diverging Pathways? Palliative Care in Cancer and in Heart Failure

Evidence and education have helped to normalize early, integrated palliative care approaches and improve outcomes for patients with advanced cancer.[23,24] Because of a dearth of evidence in the cardiology literature, heart failure guidelines and consensus statements have partially relied on cancer care studies to recommend best practices for treating patients at end of life.[4,22] However, despite similar or worse symptom burden, depression, and spiritual well-being for patients with advanced heart failure compared with those with advanced cancer,[25] heart failure has been associated with less access to palliative care and use of hospice, and higher rates of resource use and aggressive treatment.[26,27] This disparity highlights a need to better inform providers and patients of options for progressive and end-of-life heart failure.

Some clinicians have noted that translating the model of palliative cancer care to heart failure may not be feasible or appropriate, given a less predictable course of disease progression and less well-defined transition stages by which to time interventions.[22] Even so, evidence-based cancer care provides a foundation from which integrated palliative heart failure care can expand. For example, the ENABLE: CHF-PC (Educate, Nurture, Advise, Before Life Ends: Comprehensive Heart Care for Patients and Caregivers) trial (see **Table 1**) evolved from a series of successful palliative cancer care trials, and its recently published feasibility pilot results were promising.[11]

THE LOGISTICS OF TEAM-BASED PALLIATIVE CARE IN HEART FAILURE
Who Makes up the Clinical Palliative Care Team?

Various health care providers from multiple fields comprise the clinical component of a multidisciplinary palliative care team, along with patients and caregivers (**Fig. 2**). The 3 main specialties are primary care, cardiology, and palliative care, each represented by various physicians, advanced practitioners, and nurses. A collaborative interface between these specialties leads to improved communication and understanding of patients' goals, more streamlined referrals to specialists, and better end-of-life experiences.[28] Interdisciplinary care increases prescriptions for symptom control medication and decreases hospitalizations, length of stay, and cost of care.[7] These 3 specialties should constitute the core of the patient's heart failure medical home. Each specialty may take a more central role in coordination of patient care at different times in the disease span (**Fig. 3**).

This partnership can be challenging because of prognostic uncertainty, difficulty with optimal timing of consultation, the desire to save patients, and the fear of failing them. Such barriers stem from an inaccurate perception of palliative care as synonymous with hospice.[29,30] Palliative care should not be seen as giving up or accepting death, but as 1 component of a collaborative, supportive approach to patient care (**Box 1**).

Table 1
Selected clinical trials and intervention studies of team-based palliative care in heart failure

Study	Study Type	Setting/Subject	Provider Training	Intervention Domains	Intervention Components	Intervention Development	Team Liaison	Team members	Outcomes/Results
Aiken et al,[8] 2006	Prospective, Single Center, Randomized Controlled Trial	Home-based COPD, NYHA IIIb/IV HF prognosis ≤2 y n = 190 (129 HF) 100 cases (67 HF) 90 controls (62 HF)	• Members chosen for EOLC/ chronic disease care experience • 2 wk training session • Ongoing monthly presentations by experts on specific topics	• Disease/Symptom Management • Self-care/ knowledge of Illness/ Resources • Preparation for EOLC/ACP • Physical/Mental Functioning • Utilization of Medical Services	PhoenixCare Model • Average 1 to 6 home/clinic/ phone care visits per month • Scheduled team meetings, referrals as needed • Unique protocols by disease & level of stability • Parallel with usual/curative treatment care	• Based on expert opinion literature regarding case management of ill adults • Validated FairCare model used for communication training	RN Case Manager	Medical Director SW Pastoral Counselor PCP Family Community Agencies	Among cases: • Better self-care, resource awareness, legal participation, vitality, physical function, self-rated health • Lower symptom distress • No difference in ED visits
Bekelman et al,[9] 2014	Prospective, Single Center, Mixed-Methods Feasibility Pilot	Outpatient HF (82% NYHA II/III) n = 17	• RN: 2 half-day workshops • SW/Psych: 1.5 workshop days	• Symptom Management • Illness Adjustment/ Depression	CASA (Collaborative Care to Alleviate Symptoms & Adjust to Illness) • 6 to 8 RN-led phone/clinic visits for symptom management • 5 SW/Psych-led phone visits for adjustment/ depression • Weekly team meetings with recommendations to PCP	• Algorithm-based symptom management taught by PCS • Validated, manualized counseling protocol taught by psychologist • Collaborative care model validated in CAD patients with angina	PCP	RN SW Psychologist Cardiologist PCS	• 1 early withdrawal • <5% missing data • 85% of recommendations implemented • All recognized depression treated • Patients reported positive experience, requested more program flexibility

(continued on next page)

481

Table 1 (*continued*)

Study	Study Type	Setting/Subject	Provider Training	Intervention Domains	Intervention Components	Intervention Development	Team Liaison	Team members	Outcomes/Results
Brannstrom & Boman,[10] 2014 (Sweden)	Prospective, Single Center, Randomized Controlled Trial	Home-based NYHA III/IV HF n = 72 36 cases, 36 controls	—	• Disease Education • ACP • Symptom Management • Communication • Goals of Care	PREFER (Palliative advanced home caRE and heart FailurE caRe) • Parallel with usual/curative treatment care, all needs met • Advanced, total home care unit providing services Monday-Friday • Phone/home visits with diuretics, as needed • Resume own provider at 6 mo w/ individual care plan • Bi-monthly team meetings	• Based on "The 6 S's," a derived, person-centered PC model (Self-image, Self-determination, Social relationships, Symptom control, Synthesis & Surrender) • Relied on data collection from Swedish nation-wide quality palliative registry aimed at improving EOLC • Care structure per ESC guideline recommendations	—	PCS HF Cardiologist Cardiologist HF RN PC RN PT/OT	Among cases: • Improved QoL, total symptom, self-efficacy domains of KCCQ • Nausea was only improved symptom of 9 studied • NYHA class improved more often • 15 (vs. 53) hospitalizations • Nearly 5× more RN visits

	Design	Setting/Population	Training	Domains	Intervention	Theoretical Basis	Interventionists	Providers	Outcomes
Dionne-Odom et al,[11] 2014	Prospective, Single Center Feasibility Pilot	Community-based/Rural HF (86% NYHA III/IV) n = 11 dyads (patient/caregiver)	• RN coaches had ≥24 h of training • Periodic fidelity checks • All interventionists in previous ENABLE studies	• Problem-solving • Symptom Management • Self-care • Communication/Care Coordination • Local Community Resource Use • Decision-making/ACP • Life Review/Creating Legacy	• ENABLE (Educate, Nurture, Advise, Before Life Ends):PC-CHF • AP PC RN coach-led phone/in-person visits • 6 visits with patients; 3 with caregivers • Uses Charting Your Course guidebook • Monthly follow-up calls for reinforcement/coaching • In-person PC team assessment	• Derived from previous ENABLE studies in oncology • Translated material to HF verbage • External advisors & clinician expert advisory groups (Cardiology, PCP, IM)	AP PC RN coach	Caregiver PCP Internist Cardiologist	• Feasible from all perspectives • Clinicians concerns of prognostic uncertainty, poor patient understanding of disease severity, and parallel PC • Patients desired earlier intervention • Small to medium effect sizes of efficacy scores
Enguidanos et al,[12] 2005	Prospective, Controlled Trial	Home-based HF, COPD, Cancer prognosis ≤1 y n = 298 (82 HF) 159 cases (31 HF) 139 controls (51 HF)	• MD, RN, SW "all with expertise in symptom management and biopsychosocial intervention"	• Decision-making/ACP • Communication • Continuity of Care • Emotional/Practical/Spiritual Support • Symptom Control/Comfort Care • Clinician Emotional/Organizational Support	• KPPC (Kaiser Permanente Palliative Care) • Home visits by RN, MD, SW, et al, as needed • Parallel with usual/curative treatment care	• KPPC domains derived from consensus statement by peer workgroup of field experts on ICU end-of-life care	—	Family RN MD SW	Among cases: • No improved severity of illness in HF • More home deaths (less difference in HF patients) • Less days on service • 52% decrease in cost of care for HF

(continued on next page)

Table 1
(continued)

Study	Study Type	Setting/Subject	Provider Training	Intervention Domains	Intervention Components	Intervention Development	Team Liaison	Team members	Outcomes/Results
Evangelista et al,[13] 2012	Prospective, Single Center, Cohort Study	Outpatient NYHA II/II HF, hosptalized n = 36	—	• ACP	• Outpatient PCS consultation 1 wk after discharge • Phone interviews at baseline and 3 mo	—	—	PCS or PC NP	• Perceived health better in AD completers • AD knowledge/attitude improved markedly • AD completion only increased 28% to 42%
Evangelista et al,[14] 2014	Prospective, Single Center, Cohort Study	Outpatient NYHA II/III HF, hospitalized n = 42 29≥2 PC visits 13<2 PC visits	—	• Symptom Management • Illness Understanding • Goals of Care • Decision-making/Care Coordination	• PC program brochure and letter of explanation at discharge • Outpatient PCS consult 1 wk after discharge • Phone interviews at baseline and 3 mo • Encouraged to contact PC for ongoing services/support	—	—	PCS or PC NP	• Significantly greater improvements in control, activation, & symptom distress with multiple PC visits

Source	Design	Setting/Sample	Intervention	Facilitator Training	PC Components	Certified Facilitator	Caregiver/Proxy	Outcomes
Schellinger et al,[15] 2011	Prospective, Multi-site/Single System Implementation Study	Outpatient HF, referred for ACP n = 1894 602 completed ACP 1292 did not complete	• ACP	• Facilitators (RN/SW) certified in 26-h competency-based communication skills training program • Unquantified "staff time" to educate system employees about intervention/process	"Respecting Choices:" Disease-Specific ACP • Call center to track referrals/schedule interviews • Facilitated in-depth ACP interview with patient and proxy • HF planning tools to accurately document goals, values, and treatment preferences accessible in medical record	• Based on established "Respecting Choices" program, which has been validated in multiple RCTs	RN SW Referall Coordinator	• Completers were significantly older and referred more from clinics or home care • Completers had significantly higher rates of appropriate documentation of ACP and hospice enrollment • No difference in 60-d ED or admission rates
Schwarz et al,[16] 2012	Retrospective, Single Center Descriptive Study	Inpatient NYHA IV HF, referred for transplant & early PC n = 20	—	• Symptom Management • Goals of Therapy Clarification • ACP • Hospice Referall • EOLC	• Chart review post-discharge • Unstructured interviews to gauge impact of PC on patients, families, and care providers • Non-standardized tool used in which 1 PCS & 1 HF cardiologist scored impact of PC on patients	—	PCS HF Cardiologist NP SW Psychiatrist Hospital Chaplain	• Reduced pain • More holistic care (psychiatric assessment, spiritual counseling, etc.) • Patient-reported increase in clarity & continuity of care • 30% of patients completed ADs • Moderate to significant impact scores

(continued on next page)

Table 1
(continued)

Study	Study Type	Setting/Subject	Provider Training	Intervention Domains	Intervention Components	Intervention Development	Team Liaison	Team members	Outcomes/Results
Wong et al,[17,18] 2013 (China)	Retrospective, Single Center Descriptive Study	Home-based NYHA III/IV HF n = 44	—	• Resource Utilization	• Data had been collected prospectively in registry of all end-stage HF patients at site recruited into PC • Weekly to monthly home visits by team based on acuity • Patients also followed in hospital-based chronic HF management program at regular intervals		—	MD RN Counsellor	• 68% died in 24 mo follow-up • Mean time to death was 5.5 mo • Significant reduction in all-cause & HF hospitalizations

Abbreviations: ACP, advance care planning; AP, advanced practice; CAD, coronary artery disease; CHF, congestive heart failure; COPD, chronic obstructive pulmonary disease; ED, emergency department; ENABLE, Educate, Nurture, Advise, Before Life Ends; EOLC, end of life communication; ESC, European Society of Cardiology; HF, heart failure; IM, internal medicine; KCCQ, Kansas City Cardiomyopathy Questionnaire; KPPC, Kaiser Permanente Palliative Care; MD, medical doctor; NP, nurse practitioner; NYHA, New York Heart Association; OT, occupational therapy; PC, palliative care; PCP, primary care physician; PCS, palliative care specialist; prn, as needed; PT, physical therapy; QoL, quality of life; RCT, randomized controlled trial; recs, recommendations; RN, registered nurse; Psych, psychologist; SW, social work.

Data from Refs.[8–17]

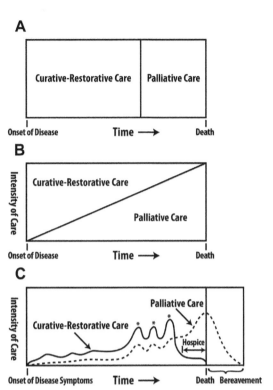

Fig. 1. Evolving models of integrating curative-restorative care with palliative care. (*A*) Curative-restorative care was previously seen as an all-or-none phenomenon, and palliative care was only initiated once curative-restorative care options were exhausted. (*B*) Palliative care principles were incorporated concurrently with curative-restorative care models, but because fewer curative-restorative care options existed palliative care was intensified. (*C*) This model shows why care trajectories rarely change at a constant, linear slope; instead, care intensity is augmented by punctuated exacerbations of illness over time.[18,19] (Reprinted with permission of the American Thoracic Society. Copyright © 2015 American Thoracic Society. *From* Lankan PN, Terry PB, Delisser HM, et al. An official American Thoracic Society clinical policy statement: palliative care for patients with respiratory diseases and critical illnesses. Am J Respir Crit Care Med 2008;177(8):912–27. The American Journal of Respiratory and Critical Care Medicine is an official journal of the American Thoracic Society. *Adapted from* World Health Organization. Cancer pain relief and palliative care: report of a WHO expert committee. Geneva, Switzerland: World Health Organization; 1990. Technical Report Series No. 804; with permission.)

However, a national shortage of palliative care specialists exists along with the proliferation of heart failure in older patients with multimorbidity.[31] Therefore, a shared-care approach is crucial. By improving clinician skills and allaying fears through interaction with and learning from palliative care specialists, general practitioners and cardiologists can be empowered to provide primary palliative care to their patients with heart failure. Palliative care could then be consulted for more challenging issues, such as complex symptom control or complicated advance care planning.[32]

Who Takes the Lead?

The role of an appointed clinical team leader, or liaison, is important in coordination of multidisciplinary care.[22] The team cannot function effectively without a clear understanding of organizational and leadership structure. Early in disease progression, lead input is more likely to pass to a general practitioner or cardiology service, with palliative care consultation as needed. In end-stage disease, palliative care specialists might take more central ownership of the patient's care. In several studies and palliative care programs, the investigators described great success in appointing a heart failure or case management nurse to communicate with patients and delegate responsibility for different aspects of care.[8,12,33–35] A single team member who acts as the liaison in coordinating primary and referral services thereby offers continuity of care, a reliably recognizable team contact, and a source of trust and comfort for patients. The clinical team leader can ensure that medical decision making is tailored to patients' values, goals, and preferences.[36]

Referrals among patients with advanced heart failure are most commonly for allied health services and psychosocial support. **Fig. 2** includes all team members mentioned previously in controlled trials, pilots, or reviews of multidisciplinary heart failure palliative care programs. Data from 2 descriptive studies on the frequency of referral types in a single palliative heart failure service is presented in **Table 2**. The needs of patients with advanced heart failure can be universal, but may also have patient, site, and regional variation. Meeting such patient needs may also challenge financial and staffing sustainability. However, although the multidisciplinary palliative care team should adopt a holistic, patient-centered perspective, not all patients require all services.

When and Where Should Team-based Palliative Care Occur?

There is no clear consensus on the optimal timing and location of supportive care for patients with heart failure, except that early and iterative intervention is preferred. This preference stems from the concept that difficult discussions now simplify difficult decisions later.[38] Nearly 20 years ago, the SUPPORT (Study to Understand Prognoses and Preferences for Outcomes and Risks of

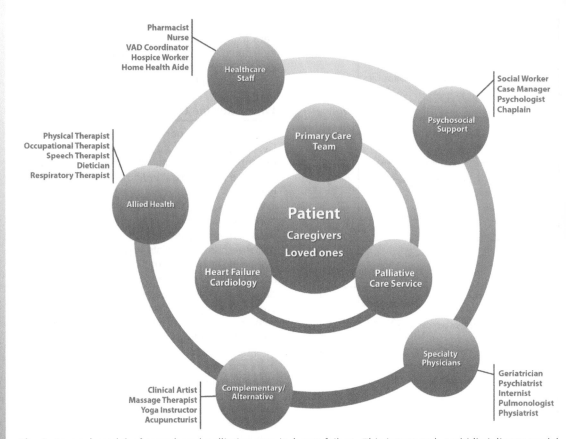

Fig. 2. Layered model of team-based palliative care in heart failure. This integrated, multidisciplinary model keeps the patient and caregivers central to the plan of care, and they are supported by layers of clinicians and providers whose support can vary over time. The core clinical team is composed of primary care, cardiology, and palliative care, with many secondary supportive and consultative services. The included providers are likely partial, and other team members may exist in individual teams to support patients as much as possible. VAD, ventricular assist device.

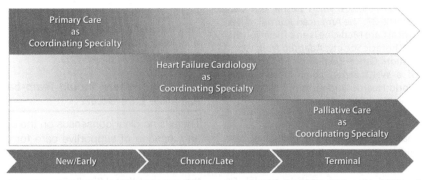

Fig. 3. Evolution of central care coordination at different stages of heart failure. In a team-based approach to advanced heart failure and palliative care, the responsibility and contribution of each core specialty may grow or decrease as the patient's disease progresses. This pattern of care coordination is likely to differ for all patients, according to their individual trajectory and needs.

Box 1
Palliative care versus hospice care

Consultative palliative care

- Addresses goals of care and focuses on quality of life, family support, and symptom management
- Can begin with onset of symptoms from a serious, life-limiting disease

Hospice

- A specific type of palliative care provided when a patient is terminally ill (ie, life expectancy <6 months if the disease runs its expected course)
- Provides team-based support services to the patient, family, and caregivers in the home or an institution

Adapted from Swetz KM, Kamal AH. In the clinic. Palliative care. Ann Intern Med 2012;156(3):ITC2-2; with permission.

Table 2
Services accessed in 2 team-based palliative heart failure programs

	Bekelman et al,[37] 2011	Evangelista et al,[14] 2014
Number of patients	50	36
Study Type	Case series	Descriptive study
Study Location	Aurora, CO	Irvine, CA
Rate of Services Used	—	—
Chaplain (%)	—	45
Home Health (%)	—	83
Hospice (%)	16	7
Neurology (%)	4	—
Other (%)	10	—
Alternative Medicine (%)	2	—
Pain Clinic (%)	2	—
Pulmonary Clinic (%)	2	—
Speech Therapy (%)	2	—
Weight Loss Clinic (%)	2	—
Palliative Care Specialist (%)	100	100
Nurse Practitioner (%)	—	83
Physician (%)	—	27
Pharmacist (%)	—	100[a]
Physical and Occupational Therapy/Rehabilitation (%)	20	66
Psychiatry (%)	8	55
Psychology/Counseling (%)	4	—
Social Work (%)	26	69
Support Groups (%)	—	31

[a] Mandatory referral.

Data from Bekelman DB, Nowels CT, Allen LA, et al. Outpatient palliative care for chronic heart failure: a case series. J Palliat Med 2011;14(7):815–21; and Evangelista LS, Liao S, Motie M, et al. On-going palliative care enhances perceived control and patient activation and reduces symptom distress in patients with symptomatic heart failure: a pilot study. Eur J Cardiovasc Nurs 2014;13(2):116–23.

Treatments) trial investigators identified substantial inadequacies in end-of-life care, but were unable to improve outcomes via a nurse-led, in-hospital, palliative care intervention.[39] The investigators suggested that repeated exposure throughout the disease span might be needed to effect positive change, in addition to a more developed health care infrastructure to support interventions. Subsequent literature confirmed the importance of constantly readdressing goals and expectations for care with patients with heart failure.[40] The need for repetition stems from the unpredictable nature of heart failure progression,[41] the ensuing difficulty with accurate risk assignation and prognosis,[38] and the evolution of individual patient preferences over time.[42] Ultimately, these difficulties might be attenuated by earlier integration of supportive care that fosters improvement in patients' understanding and acceptance of their disease and mortality.[43] Early and iterative supportive care integration might be more easily accomplished by a team of physicians, nurses, psychologists, and chaplains with skills different from but complementary to those of heart failure clinicians.

Early discussions regarding advance care decisions are preferable, primarily because they allow more time for coping and planning by patients and caregivers alike.[44,45] In a controlled trial of early outpatient palliative care for patients with various chronic diseases, 69% would have preferred the intervention regarding future plans to have occurred earlier.[46] Provisional planning can help patients avoid struggling with unpredictable deteriorations in health status and mitigate the isolation and dependency that can accompany these declines, in part by identifying resources and support in advance.[47] Early palliative heart failure interventions have been studied prospectively in outpatient[9,15] and postadmission settings[13,14,48] as well as among admitted patients undergoing their first heart transplant evaluation,[16] with varying results (see **Table 1**).

However, late referrals to palliative care are common. One single-center retrospective chart review of 132 patients with advanced heart failure receiving inpatient palliative care consults over 5 years reported an median time from consultation to death of only 21 days.[43] Late hospice referrals were associated with worse family satisfaction with hospice, unmet needs, poor awareness about expectations for when death would occur, low confidence in being part of care, and perceived lack of care coordination.[49]

Several locations for palliative heart failure interventions have been studied. Home-based palliative care was explored in multiple studies with mixed results regarding symptom burden, quality of life, health care use, and cost (see **Table 1**), although rate of death at home was higher in each of these studies.[8,10,12,17] These findings reflect the priorities of patients with end-stage heart failure, who prefer to be at home during the terminal stage of the disease, if possible.[50] The challenges of community-based rural palliative care have been reviewed[51] and tested in a feasibility pilot.[11] When rural patients with heart failure face geographic barriers to access, the importance of a team leader or liaison; telephone communication support; and definitive, concrete, end-of-life plans are vital to success.[51] In addition, although it seems intuitive that patients would prefer to face difficult decisions about their future in the outpatient setting as opposed to during the stress of a hospitalization for acute decompensation, this concept has not been thoroughly explored.

One of the best models for an early, iterative, and efficacious supportive care intervention in patients with chronic disease was pioneered by medical ethicist Bernard (Bud) Hammes at Gundersen Health System in La Crosse, Wisconsin. His program, Respecting Choices, entails in-depth discussions about advance directives, facilitated by trained providers. Discussions are encouraged with all adults whenever they interact with health care professionals, whether inpatient or outpatient, primary care or specialty, physicians or other providers. Although the intervention only addresses 1 domain of supportive care, it has been associated with very high rates of advance directive completion, higher patient satisfaction, and lower rates of health care use and costs in the last year of life.[52,53]

What Should Team-based Heart Failure Palliative Care Include, and How Should Providers be Trained to Administer It?

Several different supportive care stages have been put forth in expert reviews to delineate how the role of the multidisciplinary palliative heart failure team changes with disease progression.[21,22,54,55] From these and other studies, we have consolidated supportive care of the patient with heart failure into 6 domains and identified team members associated with service provision in each domain (**Table 3**). The expectation should be that different team members provide varying amounts of support at different times in the progression of disease, with the medical home (cardiology or primary care) and an appointed team liaison involved in coordination and continuity of care throughout.

Table 3
Domains of supportive care and team members involved in early and late phases of heart failure progression

Domains	Early Phase	Late Phase	Team Members
Physical Well-being	Life-prolonging Heart Failure Therapies (Medications, Interventional Procedures)		Physician, Advanced Practice Provider (APPs), Pharmacist
		Symptom Management (Pain, Dyspnea, Fatigue Insomnia, Anorexia, Pruritis, Side Effects of Heart Failure Treatments or Interventions)	Physician, APP, Pain Specialist, Palliative Care Specialist (PCS), Pulmonologist, Respiratory Therapist, Pharmacist, PT/OT
	Complementary & Alternative Medicine (as desired by the patient)		Acupuncturist, Clinical Art Therapist, Message Therapist, Yoga Instructor
	Exercise/Weight Control/Nutrition	Rehabilitation/Strengthening	Physiatrist, PT/OT, Nutritionist
Psychosocial Support		Quality of Life	ALL Team Members
	Community Resources (Insurance, Financial Aid, Support Groups)	Community Resources (Transportation, Home Care, Hospice)	Social Work, Case Management (SW/CM), Home Health, Support Group Facilitator, Hospice Team
		Spirituality	Chaplain
	Emotional Support, Coping	Depression, Anxiety	Physician, APP, Psychiatrist, Psychologist, Pharmacist, Chaplain, PCS, Support Group
		Loss of Control, Autonomy, Legacy Building	
Communication	Appoint Team Liaison	Maintain Open, Trusting Relationship ("Meet patients where they are")	Physician, APP, Caregiver, Team Liaison, PCS, Psychologist, Psychiatrist
	Continuity of Care		
	Shared-decision Making, Assess Goals of Care		
	Disease Understanding	Prognostic Understanding (As patient wishes to know)	
		Addressing Fears & Concerns	
Advance Care Planning	Legal (Advance directives—including living wills, appointment of alternate decision maker (health care power of attorney)	Legal (Assess Preferences and Goals of Care Frequently)	Physician, APP, SW/CM, PCS, Caregiver
		Difficult Issues (Choosing a Place of Death; Avoiding Prolonged Suffering; Code status, Considering Hospice; De-escalation of Care;	Physician, APP, PCS, Caregiver, Hospice

(continued on next page)

Table 3
(continued)

Domains	Early Phase	Late Phase	Team Members
Education	Self-management/Self-care (Adherence to Medication, Diet; Exercise)	Preferences for Rehospitalization, Device Deactivation	Physician, APP, Pharmacist, Dietician, Physiatrist, PT/OT
	Understanding heart failure and the implications of the diagnosis	Understanding Unpredictable Course	Physician, APP, RN
		Knowledge of Potentially Life-limiting Nature of Illness	
Caregiver Focus	Preserve/Foster Relationships		Caregiver
	Caregiver Agreement with/Acceptance of Patient Preferences		
		Prevention of Caregiver Fatigue and Burnout	SW/CM, Support Group, Psychologist, Psychiatrist
		Avoid Leaving Financial Burdens	Caregiver, SW/CM
		Bereavement Support	Caregiver, Psychologist, Psychiatrist, SW/CM, Chaplain

Abbreviations: APP, advanced practice provider; CM, case management.

Much work is needed to identify which supportive care interventions are most effective at different time points in heart failure progression. In one review, multidisciplinary interventions improved continuity of care, but there was little direct evidence supporting improved outcomes.[56] For example, depression is common and associated with worse outcomes in advanced disease.[57] However, antidepressants had disappointing results when used in this setting.[58] Therefore, depression in the setting of heart failure is likely to be most responsive to multimodality interventions, including pharmacotherapy for cardiac dysfunction and other comorbidity, exercise, and cognitive behavior therapy.[59] Likewise, dyspnea is a common symptom that affects quality of life in patients with advanced heart failure. An often-quoted but small pilot study described improved shortness of breath in patients treated with opioids,[60] whereas several studies have shown dyspnea improvement through exercise and respiratory muscle training.[54] Even more promising is the Breathlessness Support Service, a United Kingdom–based intervention for patients with advanced diseases, including heart failure. In a randomized controlled trial, the intervention used behavioral therapy, fans/cooling techniques, and pulmonary therapists, in addition to common treatments, to improve outcomes.[61]

One of the challenges in provision of staged supportive care throughout the disease span is a lack of provider training to facilitate holistic care of the patient. In qualitative studies, providers avoided broaching palliative care issues with patients for several reasons, such as lack of time and resources, discomfort or self-perceived skill deficit in discussing sensitive issues, unpredictable disease course and uncertainty with timing of conversations, fear of negative effects on the patient, and perception of palliative care as synonymous with terminal care.[62] However, patients mostly preferred hearing the truth, as long as they were asked permission to broach such topics, and such conversations did not take away their hope.[38,63] Strong communication skills are of utmost importance in creating open, trusting patient-provider relationships, and palliative care communication training has been shown to be effective.[64,65] Several of the heart failure–specific pilots and trials listed in **Table 1** relied on at least some level of training for facilitators of palliative interventions.[8,9,11,15] One pretest/posttest design study even validated an interdisciplinary instructional seminar for nonphysician heart failure providers on heart failure treatment guidelines and effective communication techniques.[66] As with other skill sets, providers need to develop comfort with communication of difficult content. Given the shortage of palliative care providers in the United States, structured educational interventions need to be tested to ensure that all team members are both able and willing to perform their duties, so that non–palliative care specialists can be empowered to excel in providing primary palliative care.[32]

Device-related, Team-based Palliative Care

Evaluation for potential long-term MCS represents a decision point at which a formal palliative care consultation should be considered, if circumstances allow. Guidelines recommend palliative care consultation as part of a multidisciplinary approach[5] to all patients being considered for MCS or cardiac transplantation at an experienced center.[4] Although MCS can offer extra years of life to a patient with terminal heart failure, it also creates new self-care[67] and financial burdens[68]; necessitates a strong infrastructure of provider and caregiver support; and imparts high risk for adverse events such as stroke, recurrent gastrointestinal bleed, chronic infection, and pump failure, all of which can seriously affect quality of life.[69] Several reviews have helped to establish a consensus opinion regarding the importance of team-based care of patients with MCS before, during, and after device implantation.[70,71]

During the index admission for MCS, experts have advocated a much more comprehensive advance care planning intervention. This intervention has been referred to as preparedness planning, and takes into account multiple MCS-specific factors that are not addressed in traditional advance directives (**Table 4**). Preparedness planning also requires open communication to establish realistic expectations and address difficult topics, such as triggers for device withdrawal.[72] In 1 single-center study, using a multidisciplinary approach, length of stay was decreased, and costs and 30-day readmissions were reduced,[73] but larger controlled trials are needed to establish efficacy and patient satisfaction.

The complexities of living with MCS necessitate continued team-based care after discharge. Adjusting to new limitations, fear of device malfunction, and conflicting feelings of hope and uncertainty for the future all created great psychosocial stress for patients,[74] and were associated with posttraumatic stress disorder in caregivers.[75] Successful models of outpatient, community-based care of patients with MCS rely on significant contributions from multiple team members, as well as dedication to adherence from patients and caregivers.[76] In addition, device deactivation at end of life for patients with MCS is often necessary

Table 4
Common differences between traditional advance directives and preparedness plans in patients receiving left ventricular assist devices (LVADs) as destination therapy

Measure to Be Considered	Advance Directive	Preparedness Plan
Antibiotics: long-term role	+	++
Artificial nutrition	+	++
Blood transfusions	+	++
Goals and expectations	–	++
Hemodialysis	+	++
Hydration	+	++
Intracranial hemorrhage	–	++
LVAD failure	–	++
LVAD infection	–	++
Organ donation	++	++
Mechanical ventilation	++	++
Postoperative plans for rehabilitation	–	++
Power of attorney appointed	++	++
Psychosocial assessment	–	++
Review of perioperative morbidity and mortality	–	++
Social dynamics reviewed	–	++
Spiritual and/or religious preferences	++	++
Stroke	–	++

Notation: –, not generally found in document; +, may be found in document; ++, often found in document.
Data from Swetz KM, Freeman MR, AbouEzzeddine OF, et al. Palliative medicine consultation for preparedness planning in patients receiving left ventricular assist devices as destination therapy. Mayo Clin Proc 2011;86(6):495.

to allow death. Navigating this ethically complex and challenging issue with patients calls for assistance and support from palliative care specialists.[77]

GAPS IN KNOWLEDGE: FUTURE DIRECTIONS

Although extensive expert opinion and consensus has been published regarding the importance of a team-based approach to palliative care in heart failure, prospective studies are lacking. Important gaps include the feasibility and effectiveness of using non–palliative care specialists as purveyors of primary palliative care, optimal components of comprehensive palliative interventions, and long-term outcomes associated with early and iterative advance care planning. The greatest challenge is less tangible: the culture must be changed such that all providers of health care services embrace palliative care, not as terminal or comfort care of dying patients but as supportive, holistic care of all patients. Those who treat patients with heart failure must take up the cause of treating not just the disease but the person with the disease.

To that end, the same team-based approach that we believe can optimize outcomes for patients with heart failure should be applied to optimizing delivery of palliative heart failure care. In line with the concept of a medical home that provides and coordinates continuous care throughout the disease span for patients with heart failure, many successful trials, pilots, and single-center programs used interdisciplinary conferences that met regularly to discuss their patient cohort.[8–10,78] This team-based conference model allows (1) a healthy exchange of ideas and reciprocal learning among professionals, (2) prioritization of competing treatment preferences based on the preferences that most benefit patients, (3) coordination of services to minimize redundancy, (4) mutability of individualized treatment plans as the disease progresses, and (5) streamlined communication between patients and the team to maximize understanding and trust.

Continuity of care in a heart failure medical home is not just a temporal concept across the patient's lifespan but also an interdisciplinary one across various specialty providers of holistic health care. The hierarchy of the heart failure medical home would have stability, in that appointed team liaisons would consistently provide a reliable interface between team and patient, and fluidity, in that central/primary and peripheral/consultative patient care roles might vary by individual patient and change over time. We contend that the concept of an annual heart failure review, put forth previously in a statement from the AHA on decision making in heart failure,[38] might offer the ideal setting for periodic reassessment of patients' goals, values, and preferences as they change, whether it occurs in the office of a primary care doctor, heart failure cardiologist, or palliative care specialist.

SUMMARY

Palliative care in heart failure should no longer be thought of as comfort administered to dying patients; it should instead refer to team-based, holistic, supportive care of patients across the span of heart failure progression, beginning early in the disease process, intensifying at patients' end of life, and extending into the bereavement phase for their caregivers. It must iteratively address patients' values, goals, and preferences regarding treatment, quality of life, and survival. As such, the team will change and grow in a manner reflective of changes and growth in patients during the span of the disease. A broad range of providers must be trained in communication techniques and interdisciplinary collaboration skills to ensure their confidence and ability in approaching the whole patient. How best to deliver such care will require further research to establish cost-effective, feasible, and sustainable models of multidisciplinary heart failure care.

REFERENCES

1. Go AS, Mozaffarian D, Roger VL, et al. Heart disease and stroke statistics–2013 update: a report from the American Heart Association. Circulation 2013;127(1):e6–245.
2. Committee on Quality of Health Care in America IoM. Crossing the quality chasm: a new health system for the 21st century. Washington, DC: The National Academies Press; 2001.
3. Epping-Jordan JE, Pruitt SD, Bengoa R, et al. Improving the quality of health care for chronic conditions. Qual Saf Health Care 2004;13(4):299–305.
4. Yancy CW, Jessup M, Bozkurt B, et al. 2013 ACCF/AHA guideline for the management of heart failure: a report of the American College of Cardiology Foundation/American Heart Association Task Force on practice guidelines. Circulation 2013; 128(16):e240–327.
5. Feldman D, Pamboukian SV, Teuteberg JJ, et al. The 2013 International Society for heart and lung transplantation guidelines for mechanical circulatory support: executive summary. J Heart Lung Transplant 2013;32(2):157–87.
6. Gohler A, Januzzi JL, Worrell SS, et al. A systematic meta-analysis of the efficacy and heterogeneity of disease management programs in congestive heart failure. J Card Fail 2006;12(7):554–67.
7. Grady KL, Dracup K, Kennedy G, et al. Team management of patients with heart failure: a statement for healthcare professionals from The Cardiovascular Nursing Council of the American Heart Association. Circulation 2000;102(19):2443–56.
8. Aiken LS, Butner J, Lockhart CA, et al. Outcome evaluation of a randomized trial of the PhoenixCare intervention: program of case management and coordinated care for the seriously chronically ill. J Palliat Med 2006;9(1):111–26.
9. Bekelman DB, Hooker S, Nowels CT, et al. Feasibility and acceptability of a collaborative care intervention to improve symptoms and quality of life in chronic heart failure: mixed methods pilot trial. J Palliat Med 2014;17(2):145–51.
10. Brannstrom M, Boman K. Effects of person-centred and integrated chronic heart failure and palliative home care. PREFER: a randomized controlled study. Eur J Heart Fail 2014;16(10):1142–51.
11. Dionne-Odom JN, Kono A, Frost J, et al. Translating and testing the ENABLE: CHF-PC concurrent palliative care model for older adults with heart failure and their family caregivers. J Palliat Med 2014; 17(9):995–1004.
12. Enguidanos SM, Cherin D, Brumley R. Home-based palliative care study: site of death, and costs of medical care for patients with congestive heart failure, chronic obstructive pulmonary disease, and cancer. J Soc Work End Life Palliat Care 2005;1(3):37–56.
13. Evangelista LS, Motie M, Lombardo D, et al. Does preparedness planning improve attitudes and completion of advance directives in patients with symptomatic heart failure? J Palliat Med 2012; 15(12):1316–20.
14. Evangelista LS, Liao S, Motie M, et al. On-going palliative care enhances perceived control and patient activation and reduces symptom distress in patients with symptomatic heart failure: a pilot study. Eur J Cardiovasc Nurs 2014;13(2):116–23.
15. Schellinger S, Sidebottom A, Briggs L. Disease specific advance care planning for heart failure patients: implementation in a large health system. J Palliat Med 2011;14(11):1224–30.
16. Schwarz ER, Baraghoush A, Morrissey RP, et al. Pilot study of palliative care consultation in patients with advanced heart failure referred for cardiac transplantation. J Palliat Med 2012;15(1):12–5.
17. Wong RC, Tan PT, Seow YH, et al. Home-based advance care programme is effective in reducing hospitalisations of advanced heart failure patients: a

clinical and healthcare cost study. Ann Acad Med Singap 2013;42(9):466–71.

18. Cancer pain relief and palliative care. Report of a WHO Expert Committee. World Health Organ Tech Rep Ser 1990;804:1–75.

19. Adler ED, Goldfinger JZ, Kalman J, et al. Palliative care in the treatment of advanced heart failure. Circulation 2009;120(25):2597–606.

20. Goodlin SJ, Hauptman PJ, Arnold R, et al. Consensus statement: palliative and supportive care in advanced heart failure. J Card Fail 2004; 10(3):200–9.

21. Hauptman PJ, Havranek EP. Integrating palliative care into heart failure care. Arch Intern Med 2005; 165(4):374–8.

22. Jaarsma T, Beattie JM, Ryder M, et al. Palliative care in heart failure: a position statement from the palliative care workshop of the Heart Failure Association of the European Society of Cardiology. Eur J Heart Fail 2009;11(5):433–43.

23. Rangachari D, Smith TJ. Integrating palliative care in oncology: the oncologist as a primary palliative care provider. Cancer J 2013;19(5):373–8.

24. Smith TJ, Temin S, Alesi ER, et al. American Society of Clinical Oncology provisional clinical opinion: the integration of palliative care into standard oncology care. J Clin Oncol 2012;30(8):880–7.

25. Bekelman DB, Rumsfeld JS, Havranek EP, et al. Symptom burden, depression, and spiritual well-being: a comparison of heart failure and advanced cancer patients. J Gen Intern Med 2009;24(5):592–8.

26. Setoguchi S, Glynn RJ, Stedman M, et al. Hospice, opiates, and acute care service use among the elderly before death from heart failure or cancer. Am Heart J 2010;160(1):139–44.

27. Tanvetyanon T, Leighton JC. Life-sustaining treatments in patients who died of chronic congestive heart failure compared with metastatic cancer. Crit Care Med 2003;31(1):60–4.

28. Jaarsma T, Brons M, Kraai I, et al. Components of heart failure management in home care; a literature review. Eur J Cardiovasc Nurs 2013;12(3):230–41.

29. Dunlay SM, Foxen JL, Cole T, et al. A survey of clinician attitudes and self-reported practices regarding end-of-life care in heart failure. Palliat Med 2014; 29(3):260–7.

30. Kavalieratos D, Mitchell EM, Carey TS, et al. "Not the 'grim reaper service'": an assessment of provider knowledge, attitudes, and perceptions regarding palliative care referral barriers in heart failure. J Amer Heart Assoc 2014;3(1):e000544.

31. Lupu D. Estimate of current hospice and palliative medicine physician workforce shortage. J Pain Symptom Manage 2010;40(6):899–911.

32. Quill TE, Abernethy AP. Generalist plus specialist palliative care–creating a more sustainable model. N Engl J Med 2013;368(13):1173–5.

33. Daley A, Matthews C, Williams A. Heart failure and palliative care services working in partnership: report of a new model of care. Palliat Med 2006; 20(6):593–601.

34. Jaarsma T, Stromberg A, De Geest S, et al. Heart failure management programmes in Europe. Eur J Cardiovasc Nurs 2006;5(3):197–205.

35. Segal DI, O'Hanlon D, Rahman N, et al. Incorporating palliative care into heart failure management: a new model of care. Int J Palliat Nurs 2005;11(3): 135–6.

36. Boyd KJ, Worth A, Kendall M, et al. Making sure services deliver for people with advanced heart failure: a longitudinal qualitative study of patients, family carers, and health professionals. Palliat Med 2009; 23(8):767–76.

37. Bekelman DB, Nowels CT, Allen LA, et al. Outpatient palliative care for chronic heart failure: a case series. J Palliat Med 2011;14(7):815–21.

38. Allen LA, Stevenson LW, Grady KL, et al. Decision making in advanced heart failure: a scientific statement from the American Heart Association. Circulation 2012;125(15):1928–52.

39. A controlled trial to improve care for seriously ill hospitalized patients. The Study to Understand Prognoses and Preferences for Outcomes and Risks of Treatments (SUPPORT). The SUPPORT Principal Investigators. J Am Med Assoc 1995; 274(20):1591–8.

40. Collins LG, Parks SM, Winter L. The state of advance care planning: one decade after SUPPORT. Am J Hosp Palliat Care 2006;23(5):378–84.

41. Gill TM, Gahbauer EA, Han L, et al. Trajectories of disability in the last year of life. N Engl J Med 2010;362(13):1173–80.

42. Stevenson LW, Hellkamp AS, Leier CV, et al. Changing preferences for survival after hospitalization with advanced heart failure. J Am Coll Cardiol 2008; 52(21):1702–8.

43. Bakitas M, Macmartin M, Trzepkowski K, et al. Palliative care consultations for heart failure patients: how many, when, and why? J Card Fail 2013;19(3): 193–201.

44. Barclay S, Momen N, Case-Upton S, et al. End-of-life care conversations with heart failure patients: a systematic literature review and narrative synthesis. Br J Gen Pract 2011;61(582):e49–62.

45. Bekelman DB, Nowels CT, Retrum JH, et al. Giving voice to patients' and family caregivers' needs in chronic heart failure: implications for palliative care programs. J Palliat Med 2011;14(12):1317–24.

46. Rabow MW, Petersen J, Schanche K, et al. The comprehensive care team: a description of a controlled trial of care at the beginning of the end of life. J Palliat Med 2003;6(3):489–99.

47. Fitzsimons D, Mullan D, Wilson JS, et al. The challenge of patients' unmet palliative care needs in

the final stages of chronic illness. Palliat Med 2007; 21(4):313–22.

48. Evangelista LS, Lombardo D, Malik S, et al. Examining the effects of an outpatient palliative care consultation on symptom burden, depression, and quality of life in patients with symptomatic heart failure. J Card Fail 2012;18(12):894–9.

49. Teno JM, Shu JE, Casarett D, et al. Timing of referral to hospice and quality of care: length of stay and bereaved family members' perceptions of the timing of hospice referral. J Pain Symptom Manage 2007; 34(2):120–5.

50. Formiga F, Chivite D, Ortega C, et al. End-of-life preferences in elderly patients admitted for heart failure. QJM 2004;97(12):803–8.

51. Fernando J, Percy J, Davidson L, et al. The challenge of providing palliative care to a rural population with cardiovascular disease. Curr Opin Support Palliat Care 2014;8(1):9–14.

52. The Dartmouth Atlas Working Group. The Dartmouth Atlas of Health Care. Available at: http://wwwdartmouthatlas.org/. Accessed December 12, 2014.

53. Kirchhoff KT, Hammes BJ, Kehl KA, et al. Effect of a disease-specific advance care planning intervention on end-of-life care. J Am Geriatr Soc 2012;60(5): 946–50.

54. Goodlin SJ. Palliative care in congestive heart failure. J Am Coll Cardiol 2009;54(5):386–96.

55. Morrison RS, Meier DE. Clinical practice. Palliative care. N Engl J Med 2004;350(25):2582–90.

56. Lorenz KA, Lynn J, Dy SM, et al. Evidence for improving palliative care at the end of life: a systematic review. Ann Intern Med 2008;148(2):147–59.

57. Rutledge T, Reis VA, Linke SE, et al. Depression in heart failure a meta-analytic review of prevalence, intervention effects, and associations with clinical outcomes. J Am Coll Cardiol 2006;48(8): 1527–37.

58. Glassman AH, O'Connor CM, Califf RM, et al. Sertraline treatment of major depression in patients with acute MI or unstable angina. J Am Med Assoc 2002;288(6):701–9.

59. Rustad JK, Stern TA, Hebert KA, et al. Diagnosis and treatment of depression in patients with congestive heart failure: a review of the literature. Prim Care Companion CNS Disord 2013;15(4) [pii:PCC. 13r01511].

60. Johnson MJ, McDonagh TA, Harkness A, et al. Morphine for the relief of breathlessness in patients with chronic heart failure–a pilot study. Eur J Heart Fail 2002;4(6):753–6.

61. Higginson IJ, Bausewein C, Reilly CC, et al. An integrated palliative and respiratory care service for patients with advanced disease and refractory breathlessness: a randomised controlled trial. Lancet Respir Med 2014;2600(14):70226–7.

62. Ahluwalia SC, Levin JR, Lorenz KA, et al. "There's no cure for this condition": how physicians discuss advance care planning in heart failure. Patient Educ Couns 2013;91(2):200–5.

63. Hancock K, Clayton JM, Parker SM, et al. Truth-telling in discussing prognosis in advanced life-limiting illnesses: a systematic review. Palliat Med 2007;21(6):507–17.

64. Gelfman LP, Lindenberger E, Fernandez H, et al. The effectiveness of the Geritalk communication skills course: a real-time assessment of skill acquisition and deliberate practice. J Pain Symptom Manage 2014;48(4):738–44.e1–6.

65. Schell JO, Green JA, Tulsky JA, et al. Communication skills training for dialysis decision-making and end-of-life care in nephrology. Clin J Am Soc Nephrol 2013;8(4):675–80.

66. Zapka JG, Hennessy W, Lin Y, et al. An interdisciplinary workshop to improve palliative care: advanced heart failure–clinical guidelines and healing words. Palliat Support Care 2006;4(1):37–46.

67. Casida J, Peters R, Magnan M. Self-care demands of persons living with an implantable left-ventricular assist device. Res Theory Nurs Pract 2009;23(4): 279–93.

68. Bieniarz MC, Delgado R. The financial burden of destination left ventricular assist device therapy: who and when? Curr Cardiol Rep 2007;9(3):194–9.

69. Kirklin JK, Naftel DC, Pagani FD, et al. Sixth INTERMACS annual report: a 10,000-patient database. J Heart Lung Transplant 2014;33(6):555–64.

70. Goldstein NE, May CW, Meier DE. Comprehensive care for mechanical circulatory support: a new frontier for synergy with palliative care. Circ Heart Fail 2011;4(4):519–27.

71. Swetz KM, Ottenberg AL, Freeman MR, et al. Palliative care and end-of-life issues in patients treated with left ventricular assist devices as destination therapy. Curr Heart Fail Rep 2011;8(3):212–8.

72. Mueller PS, Swetz KM, Freeman MR, et al. Ethical analysis of withdrawing ventricular assist device support. Mayo Clin Proc 2010;85(9):791–7.

73. Murray MA, Osaki S, Edwards NM, et al. Multidisciplinary approach decreases length of stay and reduces cost for ventricular assist device therapy. Interact Cardiovasc Thorac Surg 2009;8(1):84–8.

74. MacIver J, Ross HJ. Withdrawal of ventricular assist device support. J Palliat Care 2005;21(3): 151–6.

75. Heilmann C, Kuijpers N, Beyersdorf F, et al. Supportive psychotherapy for patients with heart transplantation or ventricular assist devices. Eur J Cardiothorac Surg 2011;39(4):e44–50.

76. Wilson SR, Givertz MM, Stewart GC, et al. Ventricular assist devices the challenges of outpatient management. J Am Coll Cardiol 2009;54(18): 1647–59.

77. Brush S, Budge D, Alharethi R, et al. End-of-life decision making and implementation in recipients of a destination left ventricular assist device. J Heart Lung Transplant 2010;29(12): 1337–41.

78. Mitchell G, Zhang J, Burridge L, et al. Case conferences between general practitioners and specialist teams to plan end of life care of people with end stage heart failure and lung disease: an exploratory pilot study. BMC Palliat Care 2014;13:24.

Assessing the Quality and Comparative Effectiveness of Team-Based Care for Heart Failure
Who, What, Where, When, and How

Lauren B. Cooper, MD, Adrian F. Hernandez, MD, MHS*

KEYWORDS

- Heart failure • Multidisciplinary care • Team-based care • Quality

KEY POINTS

- Goals of multidisciplinary care in heart failure (HF) include improving clinical outcomes, managing patient symptoms, and reducing health care costs.
- Providers in a multidisciplinary team include HF cardiologists and nurses, other health care providers, pharmacists, and ancillary support (exercise specialists, dieticians, and social workers).
- Multidisciplinary care can take place in an inpatient or outpatient setting, at home, or remotely.
- Multidisciplinary HF teams should be evaluated based on their ability to achieve goals, as well as their potential for sustainability over time.

INTRODUCTION

Heart failure (HF) is common and costly, affecting more than 5 million Americans with an incidence of 825,000 per year. By 2030, more than 8 million people in the United States are expected to have HF. Annually, HF accounts for more than 1 million hospitalizations in the United States and costs more than $30 billion, with expenses expected to more than double by 2030. HF-related morbidity and mortality remain high despite available treatments. Five-year mortality is approximately 50%, and HF is listed on 1 in 9 death certificates.[1,2]

Advances in treatment options for HF continue to evolve, with new drugs and devices emerging throughout the past decade. Implantable cardioverter defibrillators, cardiac resynchronization therapy, pulmonary artery pressure sensors, and left ventricular assist devices are examples of significant yet complex therapies that may improve outcomes in HF.[3–5] Because there are considerable comorbidities associated with HF, it is important to integrate other strategies into HF care, including behavioral modifications focused on diet, exercise, medication compliance, and self-care as alterable factors driving HF outcomes.[6] Nevertheless, the variety of HF care strategies creates the potential for fragmented care, with multiple disciplines spread across different settings.

Team-based or multidisciplinary care may be a potential way to reduce the burden of care and

Sources of Funding: Dr L.B. Cooper is supported by grant T32HL069749-11A1 from the National Institute of Health.

Dr L.B. Cooper has no relevant disclosures to report. Dr A.F. Hernandez reports research grant funding from Amgen, Bristol-Myers Squibb, GlaxoSmithKline, Janssen, Novartis, Portola Pharmaceuticals; and receiving honoraria from Amgen, GlaxoSmithKline, Janssen, and Novartis.

Division of Cardiology, Department of Medicine, Duke Clinical Research Institute, Duke University School of Medicine, Durham, NC, USA

* Corresponding author. Duke Clinical Research Institute, PO Box 17969, Durham, NC 27715.
E-mail address: adrian.hernandez@duke.edu

Heart Failure Clin 11 (2015) 499–506
http://dx.doi.org/10.1016/j.hfc.2015.03.011
1551-7136/15/$ – see front matter © 2015 Elsevier Inc. All rights reserved.

positively impact outcomes for HF patients. Furthermore, team-based care is a cornerstone of the patient-centered medical home model of care for chronic disease.[7] Team-based care requires resources like personnel, funding, infrastructure, and time; therefore, multidisciplinary teams should be evaluated to ensure organized, effective, and worthwhile interventions (**Box 1**).

What Are the Goals for Team-Based Care in Heart Failure?

- Short- and long-term clinical outcomes

Box 1
Team-based care in heart failure

Who are the care providers?
- Primary care providers
- Heart failure cardiologists
- Heart failure nurses
- Subspecialty cardiac providers
- Clinical pharmacists
- Dieticians
- Exercise specialists
- Mental health providers
- Social workers
- Home health workers

What are the goals of care?
- Clinical outcomes
- Symptom management
- Cost reduction
- Patient, caregiver, provider satisfaction

Where is the care given?
- Inpatient hospitalization
- Outpatient clinic
- Home
- Remotely (telephone, telemonitoring)

When is the critical time for care?
- At diagnosis
- Change in clinical status
- Hospitalization (before discharge or after discharge)

How is care evaluated?
- As individuals
- As a team
- Ability to achieve goals
- Sustainability over time

- Symptom management
- Cost reduction
- Patient, caregiver, and provider satisfaction

The goals of HF care are numerous and diverse depending on perspective. Clinical outcome measures for HF often include mortality and hospital readmissions. Although attention has focused on short-term outcomes such as 30-day quality measures enforced by the Centers for Medicare and Medicaid Services, many patients and providers consider long-term outcomes more important.[8] From a patient perspective, managing symptoms and improving functional capacity are also important goals. From a societal viewpoint, HF carries substantial public health costs, so managing these costs is a top priority for payers and health care systems.

Using a team of providers may improve the quality of care provided to HF patients. In evaluating multidisciplinary care, teams should be evaluated based on their ability to improve morbidity and mortality, decrease the need for rehospitalization, and reduce costs, as well as their ability to provide patient, caregiver, and provider satisfaction.

Who Are the Key Players on the Heart Failure Care Team?

- Primary care providers
- HF cardiologists
- HF nurses
- Clinical pharmacists
- Specialized cardiac providers
- Ancillary service providers

In both the inpatient and outpatient settings, multidisciplinary teams can be organized to care for HF patients. In addition to cardiologists and other physicians, the HF team may include specialized nurses, dieticians, pharmacists, social workers, physical therapists, and psychologists. Importantly, the patients themselves, as well as their families and caregivers, are an integral part of the health care team (**Fig. 1**).

Primary care providers are often the first line of care for HF patients. Primary care providers are responsible for making a timely and accurate diagnosis of HF, initiating therapy, and managing co-morbid illnesses. They must be able to recognize when specialized care is required or would benefit their patients, and make the necessary referrals. Even when a patient is referred to a specialized clinic, the primary care provider may continue to provide follow-up and take on the responsibility of coordinating additional care for the patient.[9,10]

Referring patients to specialized outpatient HF clinics that are staffed with trained health care

A

B

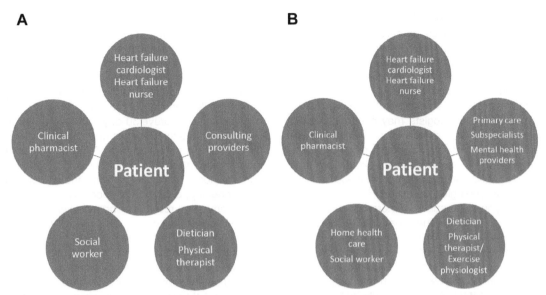

Fig. 1. Heart failure (HF) multidisciplinary care team. This figure provides examples of (*A*) inpatient and (*B*) outpatient providers of team-based case in HF.

providers who are familiar with current guidelines and available resources has been shown to reduce hospital admissions.[11,12] In addition to HF physicians, HF nurses are often included as part of the HF team, and are responsible for a diverse range of interventions. Nursing interventions have been studied extensively and have been shown to positively impact HF patient care. Close follow-up by a HF nurse in the outpatient setting has been shown to improve patient self-care, reduce readmissions, shorten duration of hospital stay, and decrease costs.[13–16] Furthermore, when the nurse-led intervention starts during hospitalization and provides assistance with the transition of care to the outpatient setting, there is an additional benefit of improved quality of life.[17,18]

Medical management is at the core of HF therapy, requiring frequent adjustments and dose titrations. Clinical pharmacists can help with education and medication compliance, monitor for drug interactions and intolerances, and promote proper medication reconciliation through transitions of care between different health care providers and different settings. Pharmacist interventions have been shown to reduce medication errors, advance patient knowledge, improve adherence, increase medication titration and optimization, and decrease health care spending.[19–24] As a result of these benefits, the addition of a clinical pharmacist to an HF team has been shown to reduce mortality and HF events.[25,26]

Outside of the core HF providers, patients also benefit from further subspecialized cardiac care by electrophysiologists, cardiac imaging experts,

and cardiac surgeons who have experience caring for HF patients. Involving dedicated electrophysiologists in the care of HF patients can increase appropriate use of implantable cardioverter defibrillators and cardiac resynchronization therapy, and allow for timely troubleshooting and optimization of these devices. Multidisciplinary cardiology care for patients with HF has been shown to improve event-free survival.[27–29]

In addition to medications, diet plays an important role in the chronic treatment of HF patients. There are many dietary considerations, including restriction of sodium and fluid, management of obesity, prevention of cachexia, and management of comorbidities such as diabetes and hyperlipidemia.[30–36] Additional considerations are present for patients prescribed drugs with potential food interactions, such as warfarin.[37] A dietician may have a positive effect on the many aspects of dietary compliance for HF patients.[38]

Growing evidence highlights the importance of exercise and lifestyle modification for stable HF patients. Cardiac rehabilitation provides a structured program for these patients, emphasizing the need for physical therapists or exercise physiologists as part of the HF team. Many HF patients have poor exercise capacity, and regular exercise has been shown to be a safe and effective means of improving functional status and quality of life.[39–43] Furthermore, regular exercise results in a reduction in depressive symptoms in HF patients.[44]

Mental health disorders such as depression are common in the HF patient population and add additional complexity, because they often require other services or care approaches.[45,46] Studies have shown that depression is associated with functional decline, rehospitalization, and death. Furthermore, there is a positive correlation between depression severity and outcomes; worse depression is associated with worse outcomes.[47–50] Cardiologists may overlook depressive symptoms and fail to provide treatment recommendations, so including a psychologist as part of an HF multidisciplinary team can help with diagnosis and management of these often untreated psychological conditions.[51]

Managing HF requires numerous services and resources, and patients may need assistance from social workers in coordinating care in both the inpatient and outpatient settings. Studies that have included social workers as part of multidisciplinary care teams have shown that they make a significant contribution.[52] By anticipating needs after discharge, arranging home health services, optimizing insurance benefits, and supporting patient caregivers, involvement of social workers can help HF patients to better adhere to their treatment plans.[12,53]

Because HF care teams are made up of a variety of providers, many facets of the team require evaluation. A team should be evaluated based on the services they provide, the providers they include, and the patients they treat. To establish which providers are most essential, teams should be evaluated on the types of providers that make up the team. In addition, team evaluations should include both individual assessments and group assessments to determine the quality of each individual provider and the dynamics of the team as a whole. Understanding that different patients will likely require different degrees of attention and intervention, teams should be evaluated on how well they can assess the needs of each patient and use the team-based model most efficiently and effectively.

Where Should Multidisciplinary Care Take Place?

- Inpatient hospitalization
- Outpatient clinic
- Patient home
- Remotely via telephone or telemonitoring

Multidisciplinary care can occur in numerous settings—in the hospital or outpatient clinic, at home visits, or via telephone or telemonitoring systems. An early meta-analysis of the impact of the location of team-based care interventions concluded that home visits reduced all-cause readmissions, telephone support improved mortality, and both home visits and telephone interventions reduced HF readmissions. Notably, the interventions that did not include a home component did not affect either readmissions or mortality.[54] A more recent metaanalysis of 47 trials from 2007 to 2013 that assessed transitions of care from the inpatient to the outpatient setting confirmed the benefit of home visits.[55] Home visits were shown to improve 30-day and 3- to 6-month readmission rates; HF clinics and structured telephone support improved 3- to 6-month all-cause readmission rates, but did not impact 30-day outcomes. Home visits, HF clinics, and structured telephone support improved mortality.

Similarly, the results of home telemonitoring studies have been mixed. Several small studies have suggested that telemonitoring can improve HF outcomes, whereas larger randomized trials have failed to show a reduction in mortality or hospitalizations compared with standard care.[56–58] One potential reason for these mixed results may be that telemonitoring strategies are often limited by patient compliance. A recent study on automated telemonitoring through implanted devices showed markedly improved outcomes compared with standard care.[59] Although self-care is vital for HF patients, these results highlight the benefit of automated follow-up, and the importance of not solely relying on patients to identify early decompensation.

These patient-driven factors may explain why the intervention's location impacts the intervention's effect. Home-based interventions allow providers to perform more in-depth assessments and discover potential barriers to optimal care and disease management. Therefore, providers are able to provide more personalized interventions compared with standardized or uniform interventions that occur over the phone or in the hospital or clinic setting.

Because multidisciplinary care takes place in multiple settings, the setting must be individualized to a patient's needs. Sometimes team members will be the same across different settings, but often teams may be composed of different individuals and different types of providers. As a result, multidisciplinary care teams should be evaluated based on the care provided and the setting in which this care occurs. Furthermore, because communication within and between teams is critical, teams and team members should be evaluated based on the quality of communication and continuity of care.

When Should Multidisciplinary Care Take Place?

- Diagnosis/new referral

- Change in clinical status
- Hospitalization

When to initiate multidisciplinary care varies based on the needs and location of the patient. For patients newly referred to an outpatient HF clinic, implementing a multidisciplinary approach to care has been shown to result in improved functional status and quality of life, as well as decreased hospitalizations.[60] For hospitalized patients, many studies have focused on the transition from the inpatient to the outpatient setting; therefore, the multidisciplinary care initiatives have been structured around discharge planning. Studies in which multidisciplinary care was initiated during the hospitalization showed reduced mortality, decreased rehospitalizations and health care costs, and improved quality of life.[12,21,61–63] Similar outcomes were achieved when multidisciplinary care was initiated within 2 weeks after hospitalization.[64–66]

In clinical practice, systems must be secured to ensure sustainability of the multidisciplinary model. Ensuring sustainability requires appropriate resource allocation, with the most resources going to patients at greatest risk for adverse outcomes and to those for whom interventions will be most successful. Because HF patients often cycle between clinical stability and decompensation, patients may need more intense care at certain time points and less intense care at others. The team-based care model should be able to adapt according to an individual patient's needs at any given time.

How Should Multidisciplinary Care be Evaluated?

- Ability to achieve goals of care
- Sustainability over time
- As individuals and as part of a team

Given the diversity of HF care teams, which encompass different care providers in different settings at different time points with different goals, there is not a universal way by which to assess and compare the effectiveness of team-based care. Teams should be evaluated based on their ability to achieve certain goals and metrics, including reducing morbidity, mortality, readmissions, and health care costs. Equally important is a team's ability to improve patient quality of life, and maintain patient, caregiver, and provider satisfaction.

Both short- and long-term goals should be achievable. Inpatient care teams may focus on helping the patient to achieve clinical stability and appropriate discharge, whereas transitional care teams may focus on optimizing care at home following hospitalization, and outpatient care teams may focus on maintaining clinical stability and timely efforts to prevent or halt pending decompensation. Because there may be different team members providing care at different times in different settings, it is essential for team members to have effective communication and handoffs to ensure continuity of care.

The ability to achieve these goals must be maintained over time. Unlike clinical trial settings, team-based care in an actual clinical setting should have no end date. Even though studies have demonstrated that the impact of team-based care may last beyond the team-based intervention, team-based care outside of clinical trials should be continuous and flexible to a patient's needs.

Teams are made up of individuals, so each person and type of provider on a team must be assessed both individually and as part of a team. Frequent evaluations can ensure that a team is structured appropriately. Additionally, it is important to determine how involved each team member needs to be for each patient at any given time; a patient may need to see some providers frequently and others infrequently. As a patient's needs change over time, different components of care will become more or less important, fluctuating based on patient status. Effectively incorporating team members and ensuring that their time is used appropriately and efficiently are keys to effective team-based care.

Yet even the right team components at the right time in the right setting may be ineffective if the team is providing ineffective interventions; therefore, in addition to team evaluations, the interventions these teams provide need to be assessed. Multidisciplinary care teams should use validated assessment tools, education methods, and evidence-based recommendations to provide standardized benefits for their patients.

When designing studies to evaluate the efficacy of multidisciplinary care, many factors must be considered. Decisions must be made regarding which outcomes to evaluate and whether the outcomes will be evaluated for individual patients, single centers, or health systems. Furthermore, outcomes can be compared between groups, or groups can act as their own controls, comparing outcomes before and after the implementation of team-based care. Whereas observational studies may help to identify which patients benefit from which interventions, given the complexity and diversity of HF patients, unmeasured confounders may bias the results. Although prospective, randomized trials eliminate selection bias, the results may be less generalizable to a broader HF population. Pragmatic trial design is important to allow for the flexibility required in team-based care of HF patients.

SUMMARY

Comparative effectiveness of multidisciplinary care is limited. Few trials have directly compared one multidisciplinary care structure with another. In trials, most multidisciplinary care interventions are compared with standard of care. However, standards of care are not necessarily uniform across trials, thus the ability to compare interventions across trials is limited. Outside of meta-analyses, there are limited direct comparisons of interventions. Overall, it seems that there are notable benefits of multidisciplinary care, but it is still unknown which interventions provide the most benefit. Different team organizations, follow-up intervals, and interventions need to be compared head-to-head to find the optimal team structure to provide the most benefit. Although it is likely that the optimal team will be different at different time points or for different patients, further studies are needed to determine which patients will benefit the most from which aspects of team-based care.

ACKNOWLEDGMENTS

The authors thank Erin Hanley, MS, for her editorial contributions to this article. Ms Hanley did not receive compensation for her contributions, apart from her employment at the institution where this study was conducted.

REFERENCES

1. Mozaffarian D, Benjamin EJ, Go AS, et al. Heart disease and stroke statistics-2015 update: a report from the American Heart Association. Circulation 2015;131:e29–322.

2. Heidenreich PA, Albert NM, Allen LA, et al. Forecasting the impact of heart failure in the United States: a policy statement from the American Heart Association. Circ Heart Fail 2013;6(3):606–19.

3. McMurray JJ, Packer M, Desai AS, et al. Angiotensin-neprilysin inhibition versus enalapril in heart failure. N Engl J Med 2014;371(11):993–1004.

4. Swedberg K, Komajda M, Böhm M, et al. Ivabradine and outcomes in chronic heart failure (SHIFT): a randomised placebo-controlled study. Lancet 2010;376(9744):875–85.

5. Teerlink JR, Cotter G, Davison BA, et al. Serelaxin, recombinant human relaxin-2, for treatment of acute heart failure (RELAX-AHF): a randomised, placebo-controlled trial. Lancet 2013;381(9860):29–39.

6. Colonna P, Sorino M, D'Agostino C, et al. Non-pharmacologic care of heart failure: counseling, dietary restriction, rehabilitation, treatment of sleep apnea, and ultrafiltration. Am J Cardiol 2003; 91(9a):41F–50F.

7. Rittenhouse DR, Shortell SM. The patient-centered medical home: will it stand the test of health reform? JAMA 2009;301(19):2038–40.

8. Department of Health and Human Services, Centers for Medicare & Medicaid Services. Federal Register, Part II. U.S. Government Publishing Office web site. 2011. Available at: http://www.gpo.gov/fdsys/pkg/FR-2011-08-18/pdf/2011-19719.pdf. Accessed January 13, 2015.

9. Hobbs FD. Primary care physicians: champions of or an impediment to optimal care of the patient with heart failure? Eur J Heart Fail 1999;1(1):11–5.

10. Konstam MA, Greenberg B. Transforming health care through the medical home: the example of heart failure. J Card Fail 2009;15(9):736–8.

11. Fonarow GC, Stevenson LW, Walden JA, et al. Impact of a comprehensive heart failure management program on hospital readmission and functional status of patients with advanced heart failure. J Am Coll Cardiol 1997;30(3):725–32.

12. Rich MW, Beckham V, Wittenberg C, et al. A multidisciplinary intervention to prevent the readmission of elderly patients with congestive heart failure. N Engl J Med 1995;333(18):1190–5.

13. Cline CM, Israelsson BY, Willenheimer RB, et al. Cost effective management programme for heart failure reduces hospitalisation. Heart 1998;80(5):442–6.

14. Jaarsma T, Halfens R, Huijer Abu-Saad H, et al. Effects of education and support on self-care and resource utilization in patients with heart failure. Eur Heart J 1999;20(9):673–82.

15. Krumholz HM, Amatruda J, Smith GL, et al. Randomized trial of an education and support intervention to prevent readmission of patients with heart failure. J Am Coll Cardiol 2002;39(1):83–9.

16. Strömberg A, Mårtensson J, Fridlund B, et al. Nurse-led heart failure clinics improve survival and self-care behaviour in patients with heart failure: results from a prospective, randomised trial. Eur Heart J 2003;24(11):1014–23.

17. Blue L, Lang E, McMurray JJ, et al. Randomised controlled trial of specialist nurse intervention in heart failure. BMJ 2001;323(7315):715–8.

18. Harrison MB, Browne GB, Roberts J, et al. Quality of life of individuals with heart failure: a randomized trial of the effectiveness of two models of hospital-to-home transition. Med Care 2002;40(4):271–82.

19. Milfred-Laforest SL, Chow SL, Didomenico RJ, et al. Clinical pharmacy services in heart failure: an opinion paper from the Heart Failure Society of America and American College of Clinical Pharmacy Cardiology Practice and Research Network. J Card Fail 2013;19(5):354–69.

20. Eggink RN, Lenderink AW, Widdershoven JW, et al. The effect of a clinical pharmacist discharge service on medication discrepancies in patients with heart failure. Pharm World Sci 2010;32(6):759–66.

21. Gwadry-Sridhar FH, Arnold JM, Zhang Y, et al. Pilot study to determine the impact of a multidisciplinary educational intervention in patients hospitalized with heart failure. Am Heart J 2005;150(5):982.

22. Murray MD, Young J, Hoke S, et al. Pharmacist intervention to improve medication adherence in heart failure: a randomized trial. Ann Intern Med 2007; 146(10):714–25.

23. Bouvy ML, Heerdink ER, Urquhart J, et al. Effect of a pharmacist-led intervention on diuretic compliance in heart failure patients: a randomized controlled study. J Card Fail 2003;9(5):404–11.

24. Luzier AB, Forrest A, Feuerstein SG, et al. Containment of heart failure hospitalizations and cost by angiotensin-converting enzyme inhibitor dosage optimization. Am J Cardiol 2000;86(5):519–23.

25. Gattis WA, Hasselblad V, Whellan DJ, et al. Reduction in heart failure events by the addition of a clinical pharmacist to the heart failure management team: results of the Pharmacist in Heart Failure Assessment Recommendation and Monitoring (PHARM) Study. Arch Intern Med 1999;159(16): 1939–45.

26. Koshman SL, Charrois TL, Simpson SH, et al. Pharmacist care of patients with heart failure: a systematic review of randomized trials. Arch Intern Med 2008;168(7):687–94.

27. Swedberg K, Cleland J, Cowie MR, et al. Successful treatment of heart failure with devices requires collaboration. Eur J Heart Fail 2008;10(12):1229–35.

28. Altman RK, Parks KA, Schlett CL, et al. Multidisciplinary care of patients receiving cardiac resynchronization therapy is associated with improved clinical outcomes. Eur Heart J 2012;33(17):2181–8.

29. Tang WH, Boehmer J, Gras D. Multispecialty approach: the need for heart failure disease management for refining cardiac resynchronization therapy. Heart Rhythm 2012;9(Suppl 8):S45–50.

30. Arcand J, Ivanov J, Sasson A, et al. A high-sodium diet is associated with acute decompensated heart failure in ambulatory heart failure patients: a prospective follow-up study. Am J Clin Nutr 2011; 93(2):332–7.

31. Paterna S, Parrinello G, Cannizzaro S, et al. Medium term effects of different dosage of diuretic, sodium, and fluid administration on neurohormonal and clinical outcome in patients with recently compensated heart failure. Am J Cardiol 2009;103(1):93–102.

32. Kenchaiah S, Evans JC, Levy D, et al. Obesity and the risk of heart failure. N Engl J Med 2002;347(5): 305–13.

33. Habbu A, Lakkis NM, Dokainish H. The obesity paradox: fact or fiction? Am J Cardiol 2006;98(7): 944–8.

34. Anker SD, Ponikowski P, Varney S, et al. Wasting as independent risk factor for mortality in chronic heart failure. Lancet 1997;349(9058):1050–3.

35. Dickson VV, Buck H, Riegel B. A qualitative meta-analysis of heart failure self-care practices among individuals with multiple comorbid conditions. J Card Fail 2011;17(5):413–9.

36. Payne-Emerson H, Lennie TA. Nutritional considerations in heart failure. Nurs Clin North Am 2008; 43(1):117–32.

37. Self TH, Reaves AB, Oliphant CS, et al. Does heart failure exacerbation increase response to warfarin? A critical review of the literature. Curr Med Res Opin 2006;22(11):2089–94.

38. Kuehneman T, Saulsbury D, Splett P, et al. Demonstrating the impact of nutrition intervention in a heart failure program. J Am Diet Assoc 2002;102(12): 1790–4.

39. O'Connor CM, Whellan DJ, Lee KL, et al. Efficacy and safety of exercise training in patients with chronic heart failure: HF-ACTION randomized controlled trial. JAMA 2009;301(14):1439–50.

40. Keteyian SJ, Leifer ES, Houston-Miller N, et al. Relation between volume of exercise and clinical outcomes in patients with heart failure. J Am Coll Cardiol 2012;60(19):1899–905.

41. Belardinelli R, Georgiou D, Cianci G, et al. Randomized, controlled trial of long-term moderate exercise training in chronic heart failure: effects on functional capacity, quality of life, and clinical outcome. Circulation 1999;99(9):1173–82.

42. McKelvie RS. Exercise training in patients with heart failure: clinical outcomes, safety, and indications. Heart Fail Rev 2008;13(1):3–11.

43. Flynn KE, Piña IL, Whellan DJ, et al. Effects of exercise training on health status in patients with chronic heart failure: HF-ACTION randomized controlled trial. JAMA 2009;301(14):1451–9.

44. Blumenthal JA, Babyak MA, O'Connor C, et al. Effects of exercise training on depressive symptoms in patients with chronic heart failure: the HF-ACTION randomized trial. JAMA 2012;308(5):465–74.

45. Guck TP, Elsasser GN, Kavan MG, et al. Depression and congestive heart failure. Congest Heart Fail 2003;9(3):163–9.

46. Koenig HG. Depression in hospitalized older patients with congestive heart failure. Gen Hosp Psychiatry 1998;20(1):29–43.

47. Vaccarino V, Kasl SV, Abramson J, et al. Depressive symptoms and risk of functional decline and death in patients with heart failure. J Am Coll Cardiol 2001;38(1):199–205.

48. Sherwood A, Blumenthal JA, Trivedi R, et al. Relationship of depression to death or hospitalization in patients with heart failure. Arch Intern Med 2007; 167(4):367–73.

49. Jiang W, Kuchibhatla M, Clary GL, et al. Relationship between depressive symptoms and long-term mortality in patients with heart failure. Am Heart J 2007;154(1):102–8.

50. Jiang W, Alexander J, Christopher E, et al. Relationship of depression to increased risk of mortality and rehospitalization in patients with congestive heart failure. Arch Intern Med 2001;161(15):1849–56.

51. Moser DK. Psychosocial factors and their association with clinical outcomes in patients with heart failure: why clinicians do not seem to care. Eur J Cardiovasc Nurs 2002;1(3):183–8.

52. Takeda A, Taylor SJ, Taylor RS, et al. Clinical service organisation for heart failure. Cochrane Database Syst Rev 2012;(9):CD002752.

53. Ric MW, Gray DB, Beckham V, et al. Effect of a multidisciplinary intervention on medication compliance in elderly patients with congestive heart failure. Am J Med 1996;101(3):270–6.

54. Holland R, Battersby J, Harvey I, et al. Systematic review of multidisciplinary interventions in heart failure. Heart 2005;91(7):899–906.

55. Feltner C, Jones CD, Cené CW, et al. Transitional care interventions to prevent readmissions for persons with heart failure: a systematic review and meta-analysis. Ann Intern Med 2014;160(11):774–84.

56. Inglis SC, Clark RA, McAlister FA, et al. Which components of heart failure programmes are effective? A systematic review and meta-analysis of the outcomes of structured telephone support or telemonitoring as the primary component of chronic heart failure management in 8323 patients: Abridged Cochrane Review. Eur J Heart Fail 2011;13(9):1028–40.

57. Chaudhry SI, Mattera JA, Curtis JP, et al. Telemonitoring in patients with heart failure. N Engl J Med 2010;363(24):2301–9.

58. Koehler F, Winkler S, Schieber M, et al. Impact of remote telemedical management on mortality and hospitalizations in ambulatory patients with chronic heart failure: the telemedical interventional

monitoring in heart failure study. Circulation 2011; 123(17):1873–80.

59. Hindricks G, Taborsky M, Glikson M, et al. Implant-based multiparameter telemonitoring of patients with heart failure (IN-TIME): a randomised controlled trial. Lancet 2014;384(9943):583–90.

60. Feldman DE, Ducharme A, Giannetti N, et al. Outcomes for women and men who attend a heart failure clinic: results of a 12-month longitudinal study. J Card Fail 2011;17(7):540–6.

61. Naylor MD, Brooten DA, Campbell RL, et al. Transitional care of older adults hospitalized with heart failure: a randomized, controlled trial. J Am Geriatr Soc 2004;52(5):675–84.

62. McDonald K, Ledwidge M, Cahill J, et al. Heart failure management: multidisciplinary care has intrinsic benefit above the optimization of medical care. J Card Fail 2002;8(3):142–8.

63. Angermann CE, Störk S, Gelbrich G, et al. Mode of action and effects of standardized collaborative disease management on mortality and morbidity in patients with systolic heart failure: the Interdisciplinary Network for Heart Failure (INH) study. Circ Heart Fail 2012;5(1):25–35.

64. Stewart S, Marley JE, Horowitz JD. Effects of a multidisciplinary, home-based intervention on unplanned readmissions and survival among patients with chronic congestive heart failure: a randomised controlled study. Lancet 1999;354(9184):1077–83.

65. Inglis SC, Pearson S, Treen S, et al. Extending the horizon in chronic heart failure: effects of multidisciplinary, home-based intervention relative to usual care. Circulation 2006;114(23):2466–73.

66. Ducharme A, Doyon O, White M, et al. Impact of care at a multidisciplinary congestive heart failure clinic: a randomized trial. CMAJ 2005;173(1):40–5.

Moving?

Make sure your subscription moves with you!

To notify us of your new address, find your **Clinics Account Number** (located on your mailing label above your name), and contact customer service at:

Email: journalscustomerservice-usa@elsevier.com

800-654-2452 (subscribers in the U.S. & Canada)
314-447-8871 (subscribers outside of the U.S. & Canada)

Fax number: 314-447-8029

Elsevier Health Sciences Division
Subscription Customer Service
3251 Riverport Lane
Maryland Heights, MO 63043

ELSEVIER

Printed and bound by CPI Group (UK) Ltd, Croydon, CR0 4YY

03/10/2024

01040374-0011